# Medical School
# at a Glance

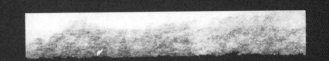

This title is also available as an e-book.
For more details, please see
**www.wiley.com/buy/9781119075912**
or scan this QR code:

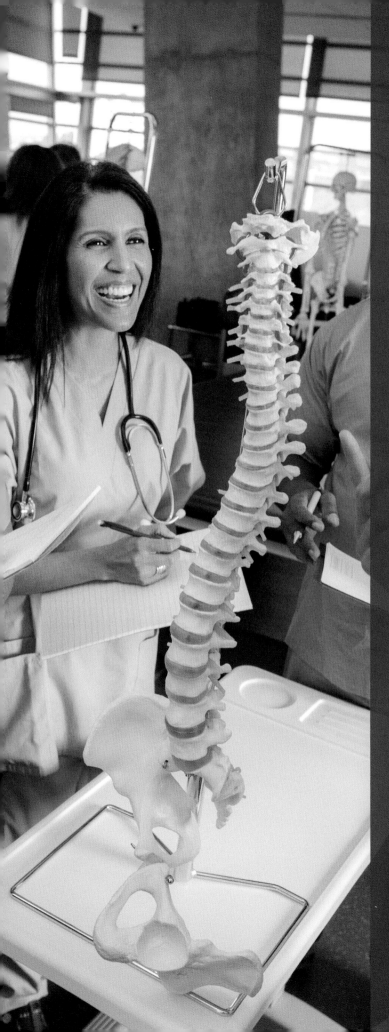

# Medical School
# at a Glance

**Rachel K. Thomas, BM, BCh, BEng (Hons), BSc**

With contributions from:

Diana E. Thomas, B.Sc (Hons), PhD
Rusiru H. R. Kariyawasam, MA, BM, BCh
Shreya Bali, BSc (Hons), MBChB (Hons), MRCPCH

WILEY Blackwell

*Library of Congress Cataloging-in-Publication Data*
Names: Thomas, Rachel Katherine, author.
Title: Medical school at a glance / Rachel K Thomas.
Other titles: At a glance series (Oxford, England)
Description: Chichester, West Sussex, UK: John Wiley & Sons,
  Ltd, 2017. | Series: At a glance series | Includes bibliographical
  references and index.
Identifiers: LCCN 2016030094 (print) | LCCN 2016030954 (ebook) | ISBN
  9781119075912 (pbk.) | ISBN 9781119075929 (pdf) | ISBN 9781119075936 (epub)
Subjects: | MESH: Education, Medical | Physician's Role | Physician-Patient
  Relations
Classification: LCC R737 (print) | LCC R737 (ebook) | NLM W 18 | DDC
  610.71/1--dc23
LC record available at https://lccn.loc.gov/2016030094

A catalogue record for this book is available from the British Library.

Cover image: ©Getty Images/Steve Debenport

Set in Minion Pro 9.5/11.5 by Aptara
Printed and bound in Singapore by Markono Print Media Pte Ltd

1   2017

# Contents

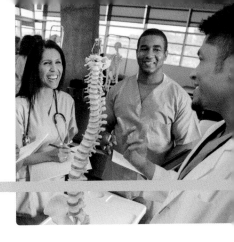

## Part 5   Considering and managing a patient   53

## Part 6   Completing medical school   73

# Preface

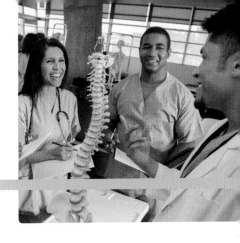

An alternative title to this book could be: 'An insider's guide to what I wished I knew before starting medical school'. It aims to provide you with tips so that you gain a running start to your medical school training. Some areas of knowledge are already 'assumed' during your medical course. These assumptions, for example about the course itself, interaction with both patients and medical professionals, and support progressing through medical school, can be assumed incorrectly. As a result, you have to learn some aspects, the time-consuming 'hard way' – by trial and error! Your time will already be a premium commodity, so minimising, or eliminating, time spent having to wonder about background issues will free up more time for you to concentrate on your studies and clinical activities. This book provides an insider's view of helpful information to build a solid basic foundation for your learning, which you can then build on throughout your medical studies and career.

This book does not aim to give in-depth coverage of specific areas, as there are many resources including other *At a Glance* titles, and the General Medical Council's *Outcomes for Graduates* (originally *Tomorrow's Doctors*) and *Good Medical Practice* for this. There are also many useful books by writers such as Atul Gawande and Ben Goldacre that can offer broader perspectives on medicine. The idea of this book is to help give you confidence, and to help you realise that you already most likely in command of some assumed basics underlying medical school.

*Rachel Thomas*

# Acknowledgements

Thank you to all who have been involved in creating this book.

Thank you firstly to the contributors – Dr Diana Thomas for manuscript editing and general contributions, Dr Rusiru Kariyawasam, for chapters on dealing with stress, solving issues, communication skills, balance and other uses for medical degrees, and Dr Shreya Bali, for chapters on behaving in theatre, evidence-based medicine, guidelines and protocols, examining a patient, assessment and management of an unwell patient, and assessment of hydration and nutritional status.

Thank you to Camilla, Hugh, Matthew, Andrew and James Thomas, and Quentin Deluge.

Thank you to Camilla Thomas, Nick May and Dr Alexander Kumar for help with photographs.

Thank you to Simon Roer and colleagues at the General Medical Council.

Thank you to Karen Moore, Loan Nguyen, Francesca Giovannetti and Kathy Syplywczak for their continued assistance at Wiley-Blackwell.

Finally, thank you to all the doctors and medical students who provided valuable feedback on drafts of the book.

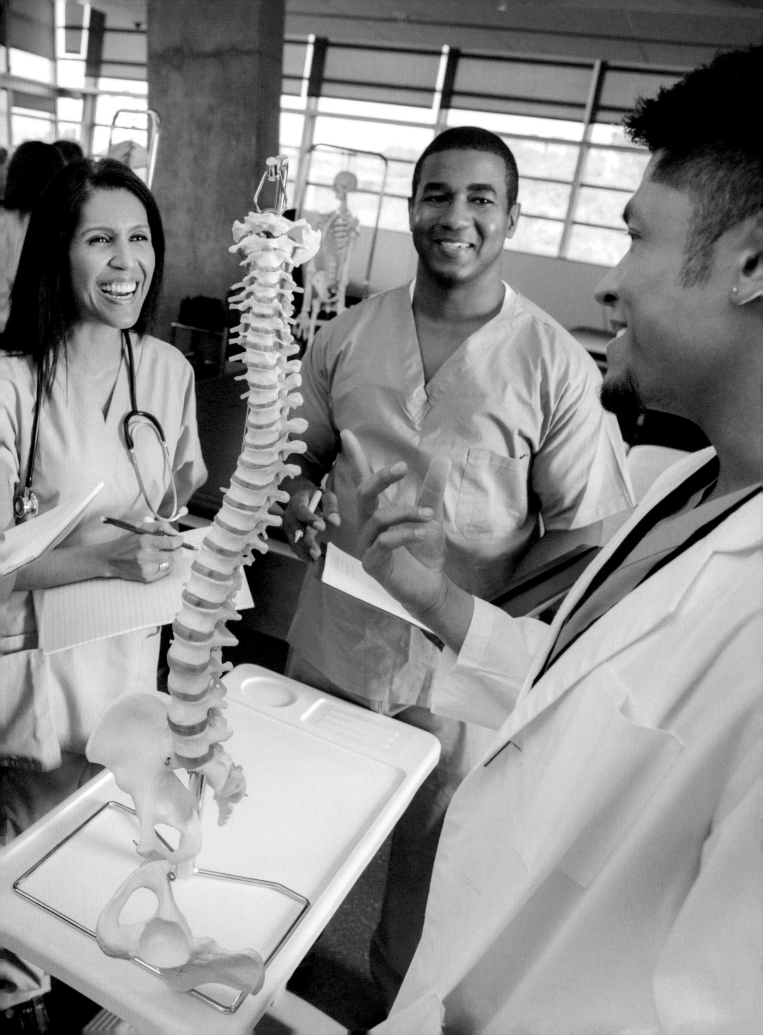

# Starting medical school

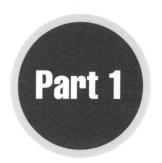

**Part 1**

## Chapters

# 1 Starting medical school

**Figure 1.1**  Becoming a 'good doctor' encompasses many attributes

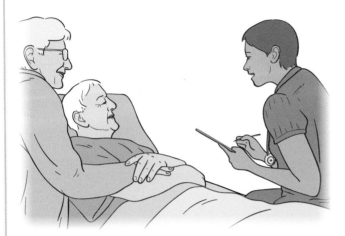

**Hints and Tips:**
- Ask for **help early**
- Remember that almost everyone is **nervous** on their first day
- Trust your own **capabilities**
- Always **respect basic principles** such as confidentiality
- **Cultivate good habits** from day 1, such as scrupulous hand hygiene

**Figure 1.3**  1948 World Medical Association modern version of the oath

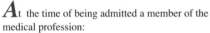

*A*t the time of being admitted a member of the medical profession:
*I* solemnly pledge myself to consecrate my life to the service of humanity;
*I* will give my teachers the respect and gratitude which is their due;
*I* will practise my profession with conscience and dignity;
*T*he health of my patient will be my first consideration;
*I* will respect the secrets which are confided in me, even after the patient has died;
*I* will maintain by all the means in my power, the honour and the noble traditions of the medical profession;
*M*y colleagues will be my brothers;
*I* will not permit considerations of religion, nationality, race, party politics or social standing to intervene between my duty and my patient;
*I* will maintain the utmost respect for human life from the time of conception; even under threat I will not use my medical knowledge contrary to the laws of humanity.
*I* make these promises solemnly, freely and upon my honour.

**Figure 1.2**  Hippocrates: the father of medicine and author of the Hippocratic Oath

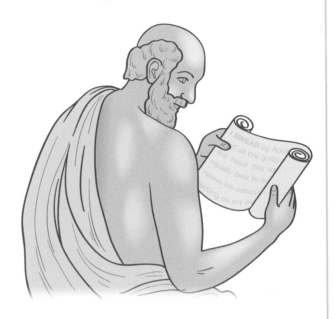

**Figure 1.4**  Some anatomical terminology

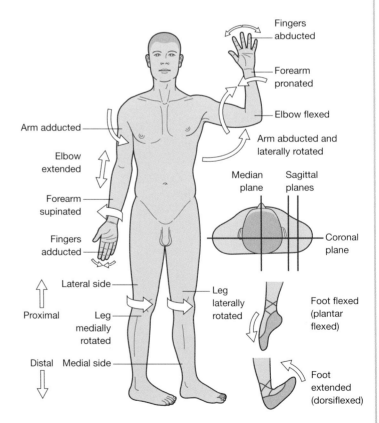

Fingers abducted
Forearm pronated
Elbow flexed
Arm abducted and laterally rotated
Arm adducted
Elbow extended
Forearm supinated
Fingers adducted
Median plane
Sagittal planes
Coronal plane
Lateral side
Leg laterally rotated
Foot flexed (plantar flexed)
Proximal
Leg medially rotated
Distal  Medial side
Foot extended (dorsiflexed)

It goes without saying that medical school is an **exciting experience** and a big **commitment**. It will enable you to meet **new friends**, as well as discovering new **social** and **academic opportunities**. As with any big commitment it can be made easier with **adequate preparation**, **well-informed expectations**, **clearly defined goals**, and **well-utilised tools** and **supports**.

Succeeding at medical school, and then in the various careers that medicine offers, requires more than intellectual rigour. The human body is one of the most amazingly robust, yet phenomenally intricate, systems in existence. So **intellectual rigour** is indeed a requirement.

It is very important to not get bogged down in the **sheer enormity** of what must, at some point, be learned. There is no denying that there is lots of it! Get used to this fact, and then move on, as past this point it is much more interesting. The learning of the facts is just a part of being a 'good doctor' – an important part, but just a part (Figure 1.1).

You may already be familiar with the **Hippocratic Oath**, which is the historical oath relating to the upholding of **ethical standards** by doctors (Figure 1.2). This was updated from the Greek text to a modern version in 1948 (Figure 1.3).

Other parts include a **strong interest** in **humanity** in general, and particularly the sick. This may sound obvious, but it is key! As you will discover, patients **tell you the answers**, if you learn to listen and to **communicate sincerely** and effectively with them. Being able to understand their **social context**, and the impact of a disease on a person's **quality of life**, is important. Being interested in **diseases**, their **diagnosis** and their **treatment** is also crucial. But it is likely that you are already equipped with these skills and interests, or medical school may not have called for you. So instead of being deterred by the sheer volume of facts, take comfort in the skills you already innately have.

At times, being at medical school is like being a detective, gathering all the hints, putting them into the appropriate order, and then piecing the underlying illness together. And there are many other areas – such as **eliciting signs**, learning the **language**, creating possible **differential diagnoses**, **performing diagnostic** and **therapeutic procedures** – which you will in time master with practice (Figure 1.4).

Different medical schools differ in their approach to learning. Some integrate **clinical care** very **early** on, while others ensure a **theoretical foundation** before you are let loose on the wards. There is no right or wrong way to learn medicine – as long as you end up being a **safe doctor**, then you have learned successfully.

## First day nerves

Usually, the first few days of medical school are like any other first few days at university – they are often spent with administration and introductory lectures. Perhaps prepare a **brief statement** about who you are, why you want to study medicine, and any particular interests, as these questions are often used to 'break the ice'.

Starting anything **new** can cause a range of feelings, from **excitement**, to **nervousness** and **stress**. The experiences are deeply **personal** and **unpredictable**. The extent that people feel these emotions, and actually show them, differs greatly.

So, if you feel a bit anxious, take comfort in the fact that you are most likely not alone. It is safe to say that many students on their first day suffer with nerves. This sense of nervousness can continue for some time. It will pass, as you become more **competent** and **confident** in your skills and knowledge.

## Types of stress

Medical school is a **unique experience**. As part of the **healthcare profession**, you will gain access to areas of people's lives that is unparalleled in any other profession – patients, who were strangers to you a moment earlier, will share **deeply personal**, and at times troubling, experiences and information. It goes without saying that this honour can cause a degree of personal stress, particularly when first starting medical school. The stress associated with patient deaths, non-accidental injuries and other aspects of medicine rarely lose their impact, but you will develop **coping strategies** over time. Aside from the stress that can be associated with **patients** and **learning**, there may be the added pressure of **financial stress**. Life does not stop when you start medical school, and in addition you may also have to cope with your own personal stressful **life events** such as bereavements and divorces.

## Coping strategies

There are many and varied coping strategies for the stresses of medical school. These will be covered in depth in later chapters – however, for the first few days, meet people, find your bearings and accept that there is a long, interesting, winding path ahead in your career, a career that is simply like no other.

Start to enjoy the **independence, choice** and **freedom** that can come with starting a course at university, and become familiar with the various **extracurricular activities** and **societies** that exist. These will help you cope with stresses, and make your time at university more enjoyable in many respects.

## General advice

Never be afraid to ask for help. Everyone had to learn once, and your seniors, your colleagues and your peers all know this, and thus will usually be happy to help. It is preferable to **ask for help early** – as often 'a stitch in time, saves nine'.

Trust your own **capabilities**, and never feel pressured into performing a task that you do not feel capable of doing. Even if the task seems basic to someone else, it is important to have enough **confidence** in yourself to know both your capabilities, and your **limitations**. You will always have both, the important skill is recognising where the line lies between the two!

As will be covered in the following chapters, ensure you adhere to important common principles from your first day at medical school – including fully and correctly identify the patient, and respect their confidentiality. You are a doctor in training, and one day soon it will be you on the ward helping these patients. Start cultivating the habits you will require in your career – from adequate hand hygiene to thoroughly documenting actions and interactions – so that these will be second nature once you are actually working as a doctor. Start learning by looking at guidelines and protocols, and embrace **primary literature** and **best current practice** to help your learning.

As with any new skill, there is no substitute for **practice**. The fact that it is referred to as the 'practice' of medicine really gives this one away! While 'practice makes perfect', perfection is, at times, impossible to attain in medicine – what you can achieve, though, is the reliable and consistent delivery of **superior quality care** to your patients.

# 2 Medicine and surgery

Figure 2.1  Some common medical and surgical specialities

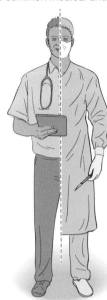

**Medicine**

- Acute medicine
- Cardiology
- Immunology
- Clinical genetics
- Dermatology
- Endocrinology
- Gastroenterology
- Geriatrics
- Infectious diseases
- Neurology
- Respiratory
- Rheumatology

**Surgery**

- General surgery
- Cardiothoracic surgery
- Neurosurgery
- Otorhinolaryngology
- Paediatric surgery
- Plastic surgery
- Trauma and orthopaedic surgery
- Urology
- Oral and maxillofacial surgery
- Vascular surgery

## Did you know?

The **GMC duties** for a doctor fall into **4 categories**:
- Knowledge, skills and performance
- Safety and quality
- Communication, partnership and teamwork
- Maintaining trust

Ensure you are familiar with these at http://www.gmc-uk.org, as you are 'personally accountable for your professional actions'

## Hints and Tips:

- **Keep an open mind** with regards to specialties – your preferences will change with experience, so don't feel you have to decide on day one of medical school!
- Try to spend time in theatre, in clinics and on the wards, as each area will help with learning in the other areas
- Consider if you really want patients to see your **holiday photos online**…!

Figure 2.2  The GMC Professionalism in Action

1. Patients need good doctors. Good doctors make the care of their patients their first concern: they are competent, keep their knowledge and skills up to date, establish and maintain good relationships with patients and colleagues, are honest and trustworthy, and act with integrity and within the law.

2. Good doctors work in partnership with patients and respect their rights to privacy and dignity. They treat each patient as an individual. They do their best to make sure all patients receive good care and treatment that will support them to live as well as possible, whatever their illness or disability.

3. Good medical practice describes what is expected of all doctors registered with the General Medical Council (GMC). It is your responsibility to be familiar with good medical practice and the explanatory guidance which supports it, and to follow the guidance they contain.

4. You must use your judgement in applying the principles to the various situations you will face as a doctor, whether or not you hold a licence to practise, whatever field of medicine you work in, and whether or not you routinely see patients. You must be prepared to explain and justify your decisions and actions.

5. In good medical practice, we use the terms 'you must' and 'you should' in the following ways:
   - 'You must' is used for an overriding duty or principle
   - 'You should' is used when we are providing an explanation of how you will meet the overriding duty
   - 'You should' is also used where the duty or principle will not apply in all situations or circumstances, or where there are factors outside your control that affect whether or how you can follow the guidance

6. To maintain your licence to practise, you must demonstrate, through the revalidation process, that you work in line with the principles and values set out in this guidance. Serious or persistent failure to follow this guidance will put your registration at risk.

Source: http://www.gmc-uk.org

*Medical School at a Glance*, First Edition. Rachel K. Thomas © 2017 John Wiley & Sons, Ltd. Published 2017 by John Wiley & Sons, Ltd.

When graduating from medical school, you generally graduate with a **Bachelor of Medicine** (BM), and a **Bachelor of Surgery** (BS). Depending upon the institution, this may be a BMBS, BMBCh (from the Latin, *Baccalaureus Chirurgiae*) or various other professional awards. While named as two degrees, they are generally awarded as one degree.

The **specialties** are divided into medical or surgical specialties (Figure 2.1). Early training is split between the two areas roughly evenly, and then commitment to a specialty naturally leads to practising more of this area. There are generalists in each area – general practitioners (GPs) and general surgeons. These generalists may also have an area of **special interest**, such as a GP with a special interest in Dermatology.

Specialties such as Cardiology, Gastroenterology and Neurology are **medical specialties**. Generally, the medical specialties start their day at 09.00 hours, and have longer ward rounds.

Specialties such as Urology, Otorhinolaryngology (ENT) and Trauma and Orthopaedics (T&O) are **surgical specialties**. Generally, the surgical specialties start their day at 08.00 hours, and have shorter ward rounds, as the consultants and team members are required in theatre.

There is often good-natured banter between the **Medics** and the **Surgeons**. The uninitiated may not be aware of its existence, but once welcomed into the hallowed halls of a medical school, it will show itself as frequent light-hearted quips in lectures!

## Common aspects

At medical school, both medial and surgical areas will require fairly similar amounts of effort. You will need to learn the **theory** behind pathologies, and how to **diagnose** and **treat** them appropriately. You will usually need to attend lectures, tutorials and problem-based learning sessions for both. Obviously, medical and surgical interventions are not always the sole treatment for medical and surgical conditions, respectively.

Both areas will require you to learn **structured clinical examinations** of the patient, and to attend ward rounds and clinics. Key within each area is learning which includes **reflection**. Later career progression requires this more formally, so it is advisable to begin reflective practice in your time at medical school. The **General Medical Council** (GMC) has guidance on what is expected as both a medical student and as a doctor, so it is advisable to become familiar with areas such as **professionalism** (Figure 2.2) and your **duties** early on in medical school.

Both medicine and surgery have a similar approach to conditions. These include areas that are covered in later chapters, including:

- Correctly **identifying** the patient
- Maintaining **confidentiality**
- Taking a **history**
- **Examining** the patient
- Forming a **differential diagnosis**
- **Documenting** in the patient notes
- Requesting and interpreting **investigations**
- Formulating a **management plan**
- **Communicating** with the patient.

It is key as a student (and later, as a doctor) to **introduce yourself**, and to **explain** to the patient why you wish to speak with them and examine them. It is important that patients **understand** that they can refuse to speak with a student, and that if they do it will not impact on their care at all. Most patients, if not too tired or in too much pain, will be happy to help you learn, but if this is not something that they wish to do, respect their rights, thank them, and leave them.

## Multi-disciplinary team meetings

**Multi-disciplinary team meetings** (MDTs) are where **different members** from **different areas** of the patient's care meet at a specified time to discuss the patient. These are excellent **learning opportunities**, where as a student you can start considering other aspects of the patient's care. They also provide opportunities to learn from **healthcare professionals** who are in **different areas** from the one in which you are currently placed. These team meetings will help you consider:

- Complex aspects of a patient's care
- Aspects of a complex patient's care

and are usually scheduled on a **regular basis**.

Teams involved in MDTs vary, but include:

- Radiologists
- Specialist nurses
- Social workers
- Physiotherapists
- Occupational therapists
- Dietitians
- Pharmacists

in addition to members of the nursing, surgical and medical teams.

MDTs can help you understand **key holistic factors** such as packages of care (scheduled support to help a patient in their home) – as practising medicine is not just about pharmaceuticals and surgery!

## Professionalism

All areas of both medicine and surgery require the utmost **professionalism**, with the GMC providing strict guidance on this. Professionalism extends beyond your interactions in the hospital and at medical school. Ensure that you pay attention to **personal aspects** of your life, such that they do not bring your integrity into question or disrepute.

**Social media** sites can easily be **accessed** by universities' faculty members, future employees, colleagues and patients. Therefore consider this aspect before posting images on sites such as Facebook or Instagram. Consider changing your **privacy settings** so that only close friends can see your content, and consider requesting that friends respect your privacy by not posting images of you without mentioning it to you first. Twitter can be a useful avenue for connection with various health agencies, such as the World Health Organization and the NHS, but it is important to carefully consider tweets or re-tweets before making them. Some medical practices advise their doctors against having instant messenger apps such as WhatsApp, so ensure that you are familiar with **local protocols**. Remember that once in the **public domain online**, these comments and images remain discoverable in the **foreseeable future**. The GMC has issued guidance on *Doctors' use of social media* to help with complying with good medical practice in these channels. Not complying can create serious implications and call your professionalism into question.

# 3 Understanding medical training

**Table 3.1** BMAT

| | What does it test? | Questions | Timing |
|---|---|---|---|
| **Section 1:** Aptitude and skills | Generic skills in problem solving, understanding arguments, and data analysis and inference | 35 multiple-choice questions | 60 mins |
| **Section 2:** Scientific knowledge and applications | The ability to apply scientific knowledge typically covered in school science and mathmatics by age of 16 (e.g. GCSE in the UK and IGCSE internationally) | 27 multiple-choice questions | 30 mins |
| **Section 3:** Writing task | The ability to select, develop and organise ideas, and to communicate them in writing, concisely and effectively | One writing task from a choice of four questions | 30 mins |

Source: http://www.admissionstestingservice.org/for-test-takers/bmat

**Table 3.2** UKCAT

| Subtest | What does it test? | Items |
|---|---|---|
| **Verbal reasoning** | Assesses ability to critically evaluate information that is presented in a written form | 44 items |
| **Quantitative reasoning** | Assesses ability to critically evaluate information that is presented in a numerical form | 36 items |
| **Abstract reasoning** | Assesses the use of convergent and divergent thinking to infer relationships from information | 55 items |
| **Decision analysis** | Assesses the ability to make sound decisions and judgements using complex information | 28 items |
| **Situational judgement** | Measures capacity to understand real world situations and to identify critical factors and appropriate behaviour in dealing with them | 68 items |

Source: http://www.ukcat.ac.uk/about-the-test/test-format/

**Table 3.3** The GAMSAT test structure

| | Description | Content | Timing |
|---|---|---|---|
| **Section 1:** Reasoning in humanities and social sciences | This section tests skills in understanding and interpreting ideas in social and cultural contexts. Most of the source material will be in the form of written passages, but some units will utilise visual images and tables of data | 75 multiple-choice questions | 100 mins |
| **Section 2:** Written communication | This section assesses your ability to develop and produce ideas in writing. The task A essay is more analytical in style and focused on socio-cultural issues. Task B deals with issues of a more personal nature | 2 essays | 60 mins |
| **Section 3:** Reasoning in biological and physical sciences | This section is made up of questions from the scientific disciplines in the following proportions – Biology (40%), Chemistry (40%), Physics (20%). The level of scientific knowledge generally equates to first-year undergraduate level in Biology and Chemistry, and A level (or equivalent) for Physics. Questions are based on passages, tables and/or graphical displays of data. They measure problem solving ability within scientific scenarios, to offer hypotheses, extrapolate reasoned conclusions and identify connection between given variables | 110 multiple-choice questions | 170 mins |

Source: www.gamsat.co.uk

**Figure 3.1** Career structure for NHS doctors. Based on Raine et al. (2011)

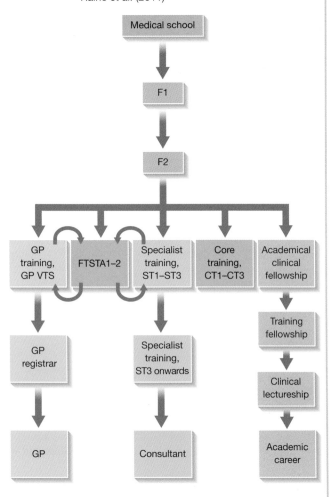

*Medical School at a Glance*, First Edition. Rachel K. Thomas © 2017 John Wiley & Sons, Ltd. Published 2017 by John Wiley & Sons, Ltd.

# Medical school

Medical school is obviously the first official step on your way to becoming a doctor. There are different types of medical schools. Generally, they can be divided into **undergraduate entry** and **graduate entry** courses. Each medical school has its **own entry criteria**, usually including independent standardised **examinations** such as the BioMedical Admissions Test (BMAT) (Table 3.1), the UK Clinical Aptitude Test (UKCAT) (Table 3.2), or the Graduate Medical School Admission Test (GAMSAT) (Table 3.3) and an **interview** and **application process.**

There are various websites, commercial preparatory courses and books available to help you prepare for the application process, as well as courses that can help prepare for the tests. However, arguably the best preparation is spending time in a hospital, and with other doctors, so that you have an amount of **experience** and **realistic expectations** of what a career in medicine involves. **Speaking** to other medical students and junior doctors about their experience is also very useful.

In graduate-entry courses the students are generally older, having completed another relevant degree before being admitted to medical school. With undergraduate courses, there may be several early pre-clinical years that are more devoted to theory, although this can vary. Some degrees are **intercalated**, where there is a year taken out to study another area, such as Business or Management.

It goes without saying that medical school is **academically rigorous**, so good grades at school in areas such as Science, Chemistry, Biology and English are advantageous.

You need to apply for both undergraduate and graduate medical schools through the online **Universities and Colleges Admissions Service** (UCAS). Within this, you need to complete aspects such as a **personal statement**, detailing why you wish to study medicine. There are various resources available for assistance in this application, as it, combined with your Admissions Test mark, decides whether or not you are interviewed. Remember that the purpose of the interview is to check your overall suitability for medical school – both your knowledge and your communications skills. Ensure that you have read some relevant health news prior to interviews, as questions on current events are common. Even reading Twitter feeds from health organisations can be a quick and easy way to keep up to date.

Towards the end of medical school you apply to the Foundation Programme (see Chapter 34).

# Foundation Programme

After graduation from medical school, junior doctors enter the 2 year **Foundation Programme**. The first year is **Foundation Year 1** (FY1), and the second is **Foundation Year 2** (FY2). These early years are usually split fairly evenly between medical and surgical jobs, to provide thorough basic training in a broad range of areas. **Full GMC registration** is achieved after satisfactory completion of FY1.

In the Foundation Programme, you will have a **Clinical Supervisor** and an **Educational Supervisor**. Your Clinical Supervisor changes with each rotation, and is required to verify the satisfactory completion of clinical activities while under their supervision. The Educational Supervisor generally remains the same for the entire year. They help you with career-planning, goal-setting and objective-meeting. You are expected to meet with them regularly, and they are your first port of call if you are having any problems. The **Foundation Training Programme Director** meets with you at the end of the year, to review your progress and determine if you have achieved goals so as to be signed off for the year. There are clearly defined aspects that need to be completed satisfactorily in order to achieve sign-off (see Chapter 34).

Towards the end of the Foundation Programme, you can apply for further training (Figure 3.1).

# Specialty and core training

After satisfactory completion of the Foundation Programme, you are able to undertake specialty, core or General Practice training (see Chapter 35).

At the end of satisfactory completion of your training, you are issued with a **Certificate of Completion of Training** (CCT). Once you have been issued with this, you are able to be entered on the GMC's Specialist Register (or GP Register), and are able to work as a Consultant (or a GP).

# Revalidation

Revalidation was created to ensure that all practising doctors are of a suitably high standard. During the first year after graduation, a **provisional GMC registration** is held. Most doctors only hold this for 1 year, although it can be held for up to 3 years and 30 days.

You must also hold a **licence to practise**, which legally enables you to work in positions in the NHS and to perform activities such as prescribing, and signing cremation forms. This is not just a recognition of qualifications. Evidence must be provided during **revalidation** to show that a doctor is fit to practise, provides good clinical care and meets the GMC's professional standards on an ongoing basis to continue to hold this.

A **designated body** is the institution that supports the revalidation, and the **responsible officer** is usually a senior member of that organisation who makes the recommendation. During this first 5-year cycle after gaining full registration, you can only work in an **Approved Practice Setting** (APS). During the early years as a doctor, these requirements will usually be met within the training programme.

**Hints and Tips:**
- Spend as much time researching and **experiencing** aspects of medicine before you apply
- Ensure that you have **realistic expectations** of medical school
- Ensure **regular contact** with your educational and clinical supervisors, as they will be your first support if you have issues, and they will also be responsible for your **sign-off** and **progress**

**Different learning mechanisms**

**Figure 4.1** Different learning modalities

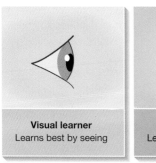
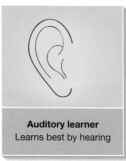
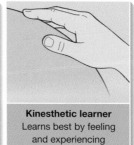

**Visual learner**
Learns best by seeing

**Auditory learner**
Learns best by hearing

**Kinesthetic learner**
Learns best by feeling
and experiencing

**Did you know?**
- Most people learn best through a **combination** of all three of the **learning modalities**

**Figure 4.2** A mindmap to link ideas

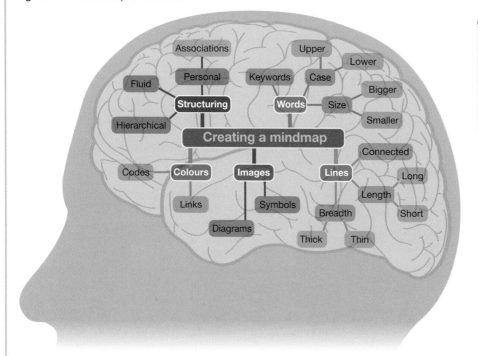

**Hints and Tips:**
- Use a **wide range** of trustworthy, high quality learning resources
- **Learn actively, not passively**
- Try to determine **how** you learn best

**Figure 4.3** Mnemonics and 'word games' can help with retention of facts

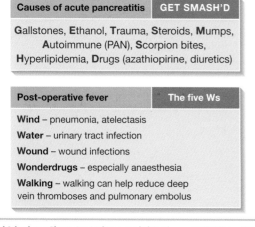

| Causes of acute pancreatitis | GET SMASH'D |
|---|---|

**G**allstones, **E**thanol, **T**rauma, **S**teroids, **M**umps, **A**utoimmune (PAN), **S**corpion bites, **H**yperlipidemia, **D**rugs (azathiopirine, diuretics)

| Post-operative fever | The five Ws |
|---|---|

**Wind** – pneumonia, atelectasis

**Water** – urinary tract infection

**Wound** – wound infections

**Wonderdrugs** – especially anaesthesia

**Walking** – walking can help reduce deep vein thromboses and pulmonary embolus

**Figure 4.4** Problem-based learning

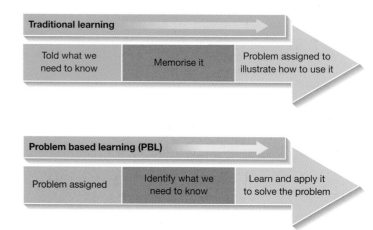

**Traditional learning**

| Told what we need to know | Memorise it | Problem assigned to illustrate how to use it |

**Problem based learning (PBL)**

| Problem assigned | Identify what we need to know | Learn and apply it to solve the problem |

Different people learn in different ways. Some learn by **seeing**, some by **hearing**, and some by **experiencing** (Figure 4.1).

Some people learn by **understanding** concepts, while others learn by rote and **memory**. There are various tests that you can do to help decipher which type of learner you are. However, reflection upon times when you have remembered things easily is usually enough. You are most likely reasonably efficient at retaining facts if you have made it into medical school, so for many people it is just a case of continuing doing what you are already doing.

## Learning effectively

Because of the sheer volume of material that needs to be learnt at medical school, it is advisable to get into a **regular study habit** of learning as you go. **Cramming** tends to lead to **poorer retention** after exams, and as each subsequent year of medical school builds on the previous one, you may run into trouble quickly if this is your main approach.

Many students find it helpful to **correlate clinical pictures** with their **theoretical learning** (see Chapter 13). This can help make the theory more personal and relevant. For example, after seeing a patient with a condition, and eliciting their physical signs, discuss aspects such as how they feel, and what their treatment has been, with them. Then, read and make notes about the condition and its treatment. An approach like this can help keep medicine feeling clinically relevant. Otherwise this feeling can become diluted (or lost) when buried behind piles of books in the library. Many people also find it easier to remember a face and their story than a page in a book – although again this depends on the type of a learner you are.

Try to focus upon learning **actively**, rather than **passively**. This can involve aspects such creating **mindmaps** (Figure 4.2). This can be an effective strategy to help solidify and then expand on knowledge as it is learned. Creating **mnemonics** and '**word games**' can also be of assistance. These can be helpful in situations where many causes or precise details are required (Figure 4.3).

**Surgical sieves** are another way of learning, which can be helpful remembering and determining causes for a condition (see Chapter 24).

**Note-taking** is something that you are no doubt adept at already. Because of the volume of material, and the fact that you are basically learning it in the hope that you will retain it for the rest of your working career, you may need to develop different strategies for this. Writing **key words** on the side of a speech card, and then expanding upon this as required on the other side of the card, can help. Dividing your note-taking page into sections so that you can summarise key words in the margin can also be helpful.

## Reputable learning sources

Most medical schools have lecturers, tutors and various instructors for guiding you through your studies.

Be wary of using 'Dr Wiki' as your main source of information. While some websites, such as www.Patient.co.uk, have good general information, other sites are not verified and therefore you should be cautious of them.

Become comfortable with **primary literature**, such as journals, as searching current papers can be an effective way of ensuring that your knowledge is 'cutting-edge'. It is also helpful for setting you up with practices to guide your 'lifelong' learning, which is a key part of medicine. Highly esteemed journals to become familiar with include:

- *New England Journal of Medicine*
- *British Medical Journal* (which also accepts student contributions)
- *Journal of the American Medical Association*
- *Nature*
- *Science*
- *The Lancet*.

Sites such as PubMed (www.ncbi.nlm.nih.gov/pubmed) and the Cochrane Collaboration (http://uk.cochrane.org) are also excellent sources of **evidence-based material** (see Chapter 11).

Medical schools have **recommended reading texts** for a reason – they are reliable, and cover the information to the required depth. Ignore any advice that your medical school gives you on this front at your peril! It can also be helpful to ask students from the years above whether they found particular texts more useful than others. For instance, the *Oxford Handbook of Clinical Medicine*, often fondly referred to as the 'cheese and onion' because of its cover colours being the same as the crisps' packet, is one of the commonly suggested books.

Some **software applications** (apps) are useful for learning. Ensure that you download those that are **highly rated**, and from **reputable sources,** such as NICE or the *British National Formulary* (BNF). Many hospitals also have **guidelines**, such as for antimicrobial therapy, which can be downloaded.

## Group learning

Many aspects of medical school feature **structured group learning** – lectures, clinical and theoretical tutorials, and various presentations. Learning to study as part of a **team** is important, as much of your future career as a doctor will involve **team-based interactions**.

The value of **study groups** tends to divide opinions. Some people learn very well in them, while, as expected, others do not. A useful role for them may be that they enable you to **explain concepts**, and answer questions, as this can really test your understanding. Study groups can also help with improving your **communication skills**, and are of great assistance in preparing for patient interactions and clinical examinations (see Chapter 32).

## Problem-based learning

Some medical schools favour **problem-based learning** (PBL) (Figure 4.4). In more traditional models of education, students are told what to learn and then assigned illustrative problems to highlight how this is used. In PBL, the situation is essentially reversed. A problem is assigned, leading you to identify what you need to know, and then this knowledge can be applied for the solution to the original problem. Even if your medical school does not teach in this way, it can be helpful to think about clinical problems in this manner, as it is similar to the thought processes that can occur when actually practising as a doctor.

# 5 Dealing with stress

**Figure 5.1** Possible causes of stress

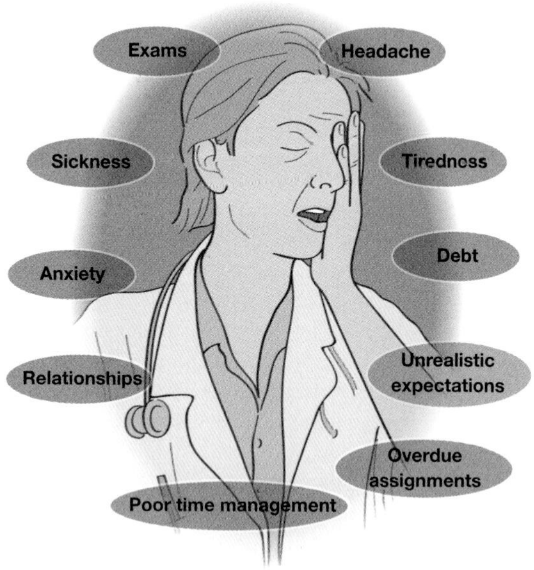

Exams
Headache
Sickness
Tiredness
Anxiety
Debt
Relationships
Unrealistic expectations
Overdue assignments
Poor time management

**Figure 5.2** Possible cumulative effects of stress

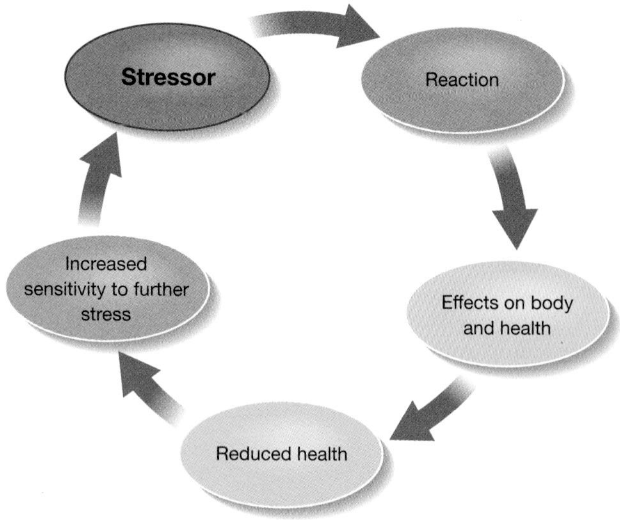

Stressor → Reaction → Effects on body and health → Reduced health → Increased sensitivity to further stress → Stressor

**Figure 5.3** Simple approaches to stress management

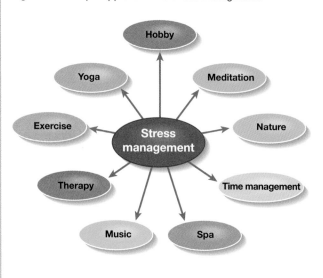

Hobby
Yoga
Meditation
Exercise
Nature
Therapy
Time management
Music
Spa

**Stress management**

**Figure 5.4** Additional sources of support

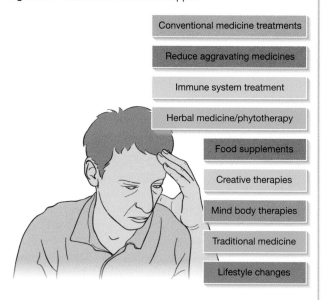

Conventional medicine treatments
Reduce aggravating medicines
Immune system treatment
Herbal medicine/phytotherapy
Food supplements
Creative therapies
Mind body therapies
Traditional medicine
Lifestyle changes

**Figure 5.5** Recognising possible signs of depression

- Depressed mood
- Loss of enjoyment and interest
- Reduced energy leading to increased fatiguability and diminished actvity
- Reduced concentration and attention
- Reduced self-esteem and self-confidence

- Ideas of guilt and unworthiness (even in a mild type of episode)
- Bleak and pessimistic views of the future
- Ideas or acts of self-harm or suicide
- Disturbed sleep
- Diminished appetite

Source: *WHO (1992) The ICD-10 classification of mental and behavioural disorders.*

*Medical School at a Glance*, First Edition. Rachel K. Thomas © 2017 John Wiley & Sons, Ltd. Published 2017 by John Wiley & Sons, Ltd.

A life in medicine can at times be stressful (Figure 5.1). While this is true of any profession, as a medical professional you will be in the unique position of being exposed to disease and death on a daily basis. This, when added to **continual academic assessment** and all the other worries of life, can make each stress feel like it adds to the next one (Figure 5.2).

Try to remember that university can be stressful for everyone, irrespective of what they are studying. **Extracurricular activities** and **university societies** can help you to meet a broad range of people and to pursue an enjoyable spectrum of activities. They can help you meet students in **different disciplines. Making new friends**, whether they are Medics or non-Medics, may help balance your social life, and may help with gaining a different perspective on your stresses. A good doctor is a **well-rounded individual** – enjoying other activities will help you with both the study and practice of medicine.

Over time you will find what works best for you when you are stressed, as there are many simple, free approaches that can be effective (Figure 5.3). If you feel you cannot cope, remember further help is always available (Figure 5.4; see Chapter 6). There are support networks within universities, such as **counselling services**, which can help irrespective of whether your concerns are academic, social or financial. There are also various online forums and student networks that may be of assistance.

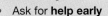
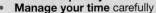
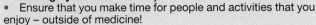

**Hints and Tips:**
- Ask for **help early**
- **Manage your time** carefully
- Ensure that you make time for people and activities that you enjoy – outside of medicine!

## Academic stress

As a medical student, a great deal of your time will be spent studying and preparing for exams. Fitting this in with life on the wards can be tricky, but careful **time management** can help. At the start of every rotation, planning what needs to be done can prevent last minute panic. Try to set yourself **small achievable targets**. For example, try to get one work-based assessment completed every week, rather than leaving them all until the end of the rotation. Similarly, **divide the syllabus into manageable chunks,** and stick to your timetable.

Consider making a **weekly revision group** with your friends. There will be more onus on you to complete the task if your friends are relying on you to prepare a topic and it is also makes work more sociable and enjoyable.

A particular area of stress for students is getting assessments completed and feedback returned. Where possible, ask for **real-time feedback.** If the assessment or feedback must be completed electronically, it can be helpful to bring up the online form on a tablet device for the evaluator to use as they assess you. If this is not possible, try to send the forms as soon as possible after the event. People are more likely to complete assessments and feedback while it is still fresh in their memory. If you find an assessment or feedback form has not been completed, **gentle prompts** such as a polite email, can remind an assessor to finish a task. Remember that doctors are busy people.

If you find yourself struggling with a certain topic, ask friendly doctors whether they would give a tutorial. **Offer to give teaching feedback** as many junior doctors have teaching requirements for their portfolios. If you are still having difficulty, **pastoral care** have a duty to help (see Chapter 6).

If you have left things to the last minute, do not panic. Reconstruct your revision timetable to **focus on key areas of the syllabus**. You often learn more than you realise while on the wards, which will stand you in good stead for exams, but it is better to avoid such a situation by trying to plan ahead.

Try to focus on your **own learning** when preparing for examinations and assessments. It can be difficult not to compare yourself to peers, as medical school can be very competitive. If you are feeling peer pressure, this can add to stress, so it can help to focus on sticking to your own study timetable.

## Emotional stress

Many people find it difficult to deal with the emotional strain that comes with a career in medicine. **Reflecting** on things that have affected you is a useful way of analysing a situation and learning from it. There is increasing focus on reflective practice in medicine and the conclusions drawn from reflection can help you if a similar situation arises in the future. If you are writing a reflection down, it is essential that you **anonymise patient information.**

**Talking to colleagues,** particularly a **trusted senior,** can be therapeutic. Many of them will have had similar experiences and will be able to offer sympathy, a different viewpoint and useful advice on how to deal with a situation.

Regularly **writing a list of things you enjoy** in medicine is a good way of remembering why you are in the profession. Write down compliments received from patients and things that you have done well. If medical school is getting you down, look back at the list and you should start to feel a bit better. Remember to keep an eye out for signs of depression in yourself and in your friends and colleagues (Figure 5.5).

If you enjoy talking to patients, **taking time out** in your day to enjoy a cup of tea with a patient and chat (even about non-medical things) can be rejuvenating for both of you.

**Taking care of yourself** is also extremely important for your mental well-being. Ensuring you **get enough sleep, eat healthily** and **take regular exercise** will improve your ability to cope with the rigours of medicine. Make sure that you timetable **regular periods of relaxation** and **plan enjoyable activities** to look forward to. Make these events 'protected times' and aim to fit study around them.

**Avoid alcohol** and other **unhelpful coping strategies.** Alcohol, illicit drugs and smoking are all false friends. They may temporarily make you feel better but ultimately they can jeopardise your health, career and even your life.

## General stress

In addition to the issues that are unique to working in medicine, you may find yourself dealing with worries from life in general. Relationship problems, bereavement, financial concerns and personal health issues affect everyone, irrespective of job or position. It is important that you have methods to deal with problems that arise in your life outside of work as well.

A **good social network** can be invaluable in dealing with stress, and a supportive circle of friends and family is often the first port of call for such issues.

If you find any of the above stresses are affecting your ability to function, your health or the safety of patients, you must seek further help.

# 6 Solving issues

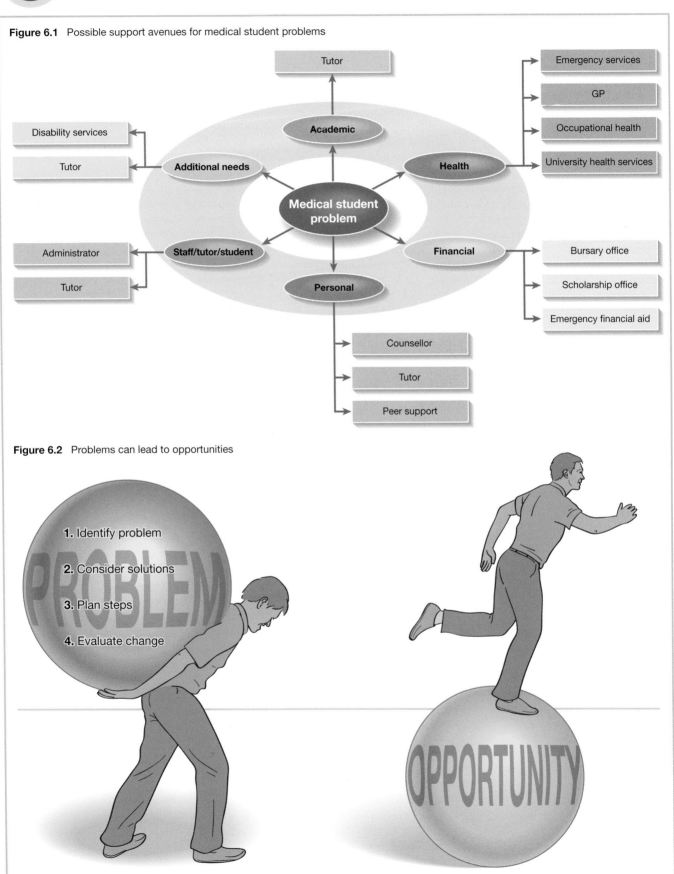

**Figure 6.1** Possible support avenues for medical student problems

Tutor

Academic

Disability services

Tutor

Additional needs

Medical student problem

Health

Emergency services

GP

Occupational health

University health services

Administrator

Tutor

Staff/tutor/student

Personal

Financial

Bursary office

Scholarship office

Emergency financial aid

Counsellor

Tutor

Peer support

**Figure 6.2** Problems can lead to opportunities

1. Identify problem
2. Consider solutions
3. Plan steps
4. Evaluate change

PROBLEM

OPPORTUNITY

*Medical School at a Glance*, First Edition. Rachel K. Thomas © 2017 John Wiley & Sons, Ltd. Published 2017 by John Wiley & Sons, Ltd.

## Starting medical school

As a medical student you are in a fortunate position as there are avenues of support available if you find yourself in trouble or have issues you cannot deal with on your own. Each medical school has its own structure of **pastoral** and **academic care,** to provide support to students (Figure 6.1). While this varies from school to school, there will be a system in place. During medical school induction, you should be informed of whom to contact if you have difficulties. This is often a **personal** or **academic tutor** – if you are not sure, **medical school administrative staff** should be able to tell you who is the right person to approach. The medical school faculty should be familiar with the system of support and be able to give you more information – and remember that you are not the first student to need help.

There are numerous ways to get in touch with the faculty. You will have been sent emails by various members, which you can **reply to,** or else a quick **internet search** will reveal a point of contact. You may wish to find out whether they have **drop-in sessions** that you can attend.

In the unlikely event that you find a particular person is not supportive or understanding when you ask for help, enquire whether there is another member of the faculty that you can contact. If you have a legitimate concern or issue, you have a right to be heard and **supported appropriately.**

There are many issues that medical students face and the medical school faculty has different people for **different areas** that require support, for example, the Bursar for financial issues.

Universities also have many different organisations targeting **general student welfare.** You can contact your **University Medical Society** (MedSoc) or **Student Union** for general support and advice. Furthermore, many universities offer **peer-to-peer counselling** if you feel that may help.

If you feel your work, or patient safety, is **compromised** by your issues, you must **inform** the medical school.

## Issues on the wards

Sometimes students find they have issues that are particular to one rotation or that are contextual to the wards. This includes ongoing difficulty performing a certain procedure or moving on from a particularly emotional case. In this case, a solution may lie in the **hospital setting.** You may wish to confide in a **medical professional** whom you feel you can approach. If this doctor is a junior member of the team, they may suggest you seek advice about your issue from a more senior figure, such as a Consultant. Staff may also recommend that you contact the medical school faculty for further help.

Members from more senior years of the medical school can also prove a useful source of support. Many medical schools also offer **mentoring schemes** to provide assistance and teaching.

## Medical issues

Medical students are not immune to **illness.** The medical lifestyle, while being exciting and challenging, can also be intense, stressful and, at times, draining. If you find yourself having health issues, remember that you have many sources of potential support available – more than people not at medical school.

You will have registered with a **GP** as one of your university requirements so if you have any health problems your GP is often be the best equipped to deal with them. **Occupational Health** is also available for medical care in the work setting and is particularly good for dealing with **immunisation requirements**, especially if you are planning your elective, and for **needle-stick injuries.** It will also be invaluable if you have to take **time out** of work because of a **health issue** or **pregnancy**.

Universities often offer **counselling services** to help with **mental health issues.** Pastoral care or Occupational Health should be able to point you to such services or you may be able to **self-refer.**

## General issues

There is a wealth of general support services in addition to those offered by the university and medical school. The **British Medical Association (BMA)** is, in a manner of speaking, the doctors' trade union. For a fee (subsidised for medical students) it offers advice, various services and opportunities, including a **Medical Students Committee** to campaign for your rights.

If your issues are serious or affecting your work you **must** inform your medical school. However, there are also a number of independent support bodies available to the general population. The **Citizens Advice Bureau** offers advice particularly on issues of debt and financial concern. A quick internet search often reveals more services and organisations than you thought possible. Help is out there, it is just a question of recognising if you need it, and then finding what is most appropriate for you.

## Problems as opportunities

Even though it may seem contrary at first, problems can often become **opportunities** (Figure 6.2).

A problem you encounter can give you the **insight** to offer better support to other students who encounter the same issue. A problem in performing a procedure can drive you to find extra tuition, and to then become **expert** in it. A problem with a fellow medical practitioner or healthcare staff member can lead you to learn new **communication** skills. **Reflection** can also be of great assistance in solving issues, and so try to include this in your regular practice.

During your time as a doctor, you will usually be required to find an area, such as one of the hospital's processes, that could be improved to lead to **better patient outcomes.** This forms the basis of a **quality improvement project.** If you come across your own issues, regarding them in a way similar to a quality improvement project can help. This **objective mindset** can help to provide perspective, and can help you to look for solutions to the problem.

**Hints and Tips:**
- Do not be afraid to ask for **help**
- Asking for help **early** can stop a small problem escalating You are unlikely to be the first medical student to face a certain problem – and you will certainly not be the last!

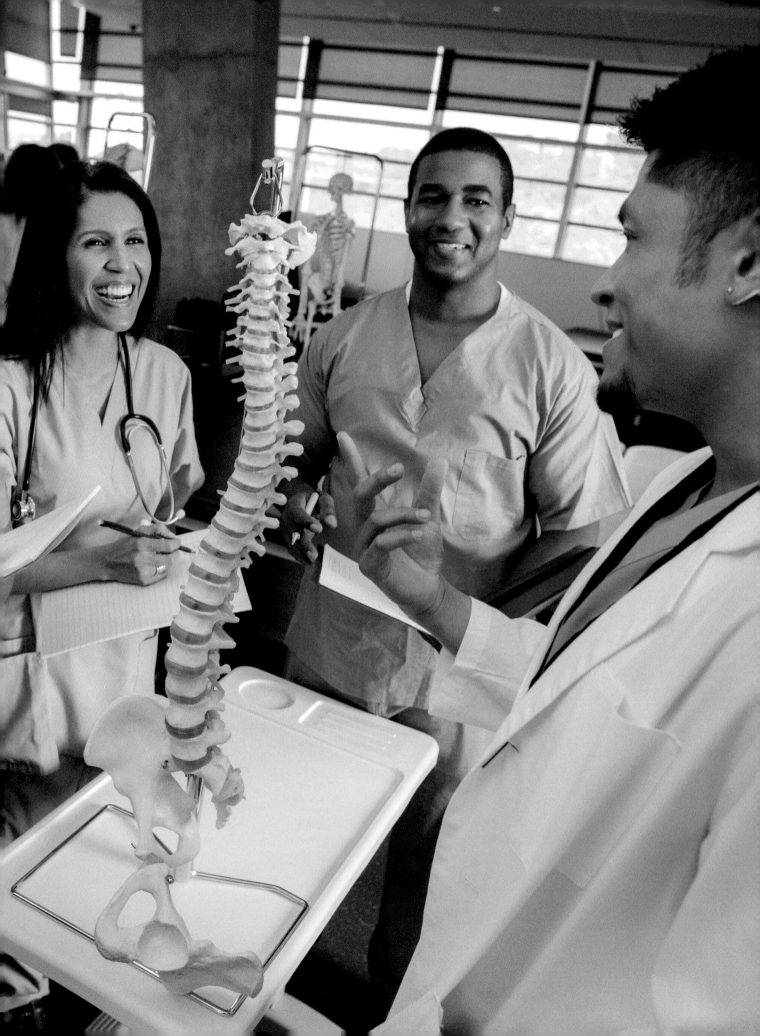

# Learning important principles

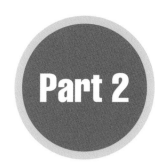

Part 2

## Chapters

# 7 Important common principles

**Figure 7.1** Six steps for adequate handwashing

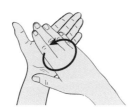

**1.** Rub palm to palm

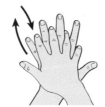

**2.** Rub the back of both hands

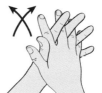

**3.** Rub palm to palm interlacing the fingers

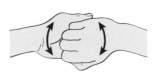

**4.** Rub the backs of fingers by interlocking the hands

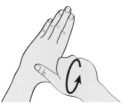

**5.** Rub the thumbs

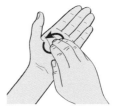

**6.** Rub palms with fingertips

**Figure 7.2** The 5 moments of hand hygiene

| 1. | Before patient contact | When? | Clean your hands before touching a patient when approaching him or her |
| | | Why? | To protect the patient against harmful germs carried on your hands |
| 2. | Before an aseptic task | When? | Clean your hands immediately before any aseptic task |
| | | Why? | To protect the patient against harmful germs, including the patient's own germs, entering his or her body |
| 3. | After body fluid exposure risk | When? | Clean your hands immediately after an exposure risk to body fluids (and after glove removal) |
| | | Why? | To protect yourself and the health-care environment from harmful patient germs |
| 4. | After patient contact | When? | Clean your hands after touching a patient and his or her immediate surroundings when leaving |
| | | Why? | To protect yourself and the health-care environment from harmful patient germs |
| 5. | After contact with patient surroundings | When? | Clean your hands after touching any object or furniture in the patient's immediate surroundings, when leaving – even without touching the patient |
| | | Why? | To protect yourself and the health-care environment from harmful patient germs |

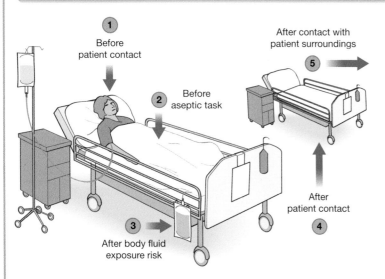

① Before patient contact
② Before aseptic task
③ After body fluid exposure risk
④ After patient contact
⑤ After contact with patient surroundings

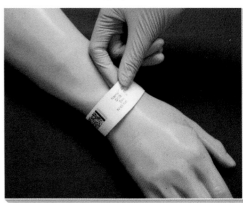

**Figure 7.3** Check multiple data points when determining a patient's ID

*Source: Figure 7.1 and 7.2, WHO 2009. Figure 7.3 Thomas R. Practical Medical Procedures at a Glance (2015). Reproduced with permission of John Wiley & Sons Ltd.*

There are important common principles that underpin many areas of medicine and surgery (see Chapter 2). These will be reinforced again and again at medical school, and can seem quite **basic**. While they are **simple**, do not underestimate their **importance**. Start turning them into **habits** from your first day at medical school.

## Handwashing

You must train yourself to undertake **handwashing** regularly. It is a **World Health Organization** (WHO) directive. The primary purpose of handwashing is to break the **infection transmission** cycle, and to decrease the **microbe load** on your hands and forearms, rather than necessarily creating a sterile environment.

Thorough handwashing needs to be performed using an **antibacterial agent** or **soap and water**. It can be helpful to carry around a small container of antiseptic gel, or **alcohol-based hand rub** (ABHR), so that you can 'gel' your hands easily. Gel alone does not remove some bacteria, such as *Clostridium difficile*. A handshake after using only an ABHR is enough to transfer *C. difficile* spores.

Use the **six steps** of hand hygiene when cleaning your hands. These are standard practice, and have been determined for 'hygienic' hand disinfection (Figure 7.1).

These six steps should be performed at the **five moments** of a clinical encounter (Figure 7.2). Washing your hands in view of the patient as you approach them can help set the tone for the encounter, and reassure the patient. While this may seem like a lot of handwashing, this is because there are many points for contamination in an encounter, potentially leading to **cross-infection**.

**Single-use disposable gloves** are part of the **personal protective equipment** (PPE) that is used to protect you from infection. PPE includes **disposable gloves, goggles, gowns, aprons, hats, masks** and **shoe covers**. Gloves should be worn to protect you from **dangerous substances**, in accordance with Health and Safety requirements, such as the Control of Substances Hazardous to Health (COSHH). They should also be worn when touching infectious or contaminated materials, blood, body substances, patients' broken skin or internal areas. Wearing gloves can act like a 'greenhouse' for the microbes to flourish in, so be sure to wash your hands both **before** putting the gloves on, and **after** taking them off.

Making sure that handwashing becomes a **regular habit** will also help you during **examinations** – when your nerves could mean it may be forgotten. The result could be a **fail** in that area of the examination, no matter how brilliant you are at everything else!

## Identifying a patient

Correct, **full identification** of a patient is a vital aspect of any clinical encounter. **You must check multiple pieces of information** to fully identify a patient, such as their:

- Full name
- Date of birth
- Hospital number

against their patient notes and hospital wristband, if they are an inpatient (Figure 7.3). Ensure that you are familiar with local and national protocols on correct identification.

The **Department of Health** has published **best practice guidelines** on identification, and decreed that **misidentification** of a patient is a **never event**. Never events are serious, preventable incidents in patient safety that must not occur, particularly if **suitable preventative measures** have been adhered to. Obviously, incorrectly identifying a patient can have serious, even fatal consequences. For instance, if a patient is allergic to latex and you incorrectly identify them as someone else, unaware of their allergy, and proceed to examine them with latex gloves, this can trigger anaphylaxis. Furthermore, the hospital where the never event has occurred is **fined**.

Remember that up to half of all hospital errors are **preventable**. Do not ever be tempted to cut corners in areas such as patient identification, even when time constraints or nerves can make this seem like a good idea.

Identification is a two-way street – remember to also identify yourself, by way of **introduction**. Introduce yourself with your full name, explain that you are a medical student and ensure that you are wearing your medical school identification badge (see Chapter 17).

## Confidentiality

**Crucial** to the doctor–patient relationship is **confidentiality**.

The GMC has **strict guidance** on confidentiality, and accidental breaches of it are regarded as **professional misconduct** (see Chapter 2). Maintaining confidentiality intertwines with the **ethical principles** of medicine (see Chapter 8).

Confidentiality is key for helping to **build rapport**, and to enable patients to have **trust** in their doctor and treatment. This trust is required to help patients be **honest** and open about their symptoms, and to enable **good quality healthcare** to be delivered.

Ensure that you **respect** the confidentiality of the patients you see. If you need to discuss a patient with another member of your team, ensure that you do so in a **private area**. If you are unable to find a private area, ensure that you do not reveal any details through which a passer-by may be able to identify the patient. When writing notes on patients for your study, or referring to patients in presentations, use their **initials** rather than their full name.

Ensure that confidential waste, such as a patient list, is disposed of in a **confidential waste bin**, or is **shredded**, and ensure that you do not leave patients' notes in public places.

It may be permissible for doctors to **breach** confidentiality in certain specific instances, such as:

- When it may prevent harm or death
- Births and deaths
- Court orders
- Notifiable diseases.

**Hints and Tips:**
- Ensure you wash your hands, as it is a very **important infection control measure**
- Remember that the **most common method** of passing infection between patients is via the **hands of the health care professionals**

# 8 Ethics

**Figure 8.1** There are multiple ethical principles involved in good medical practice

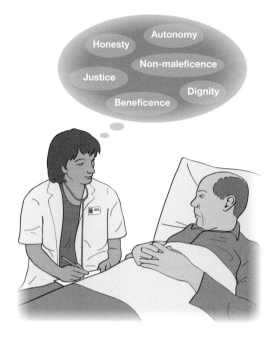

Honesty · Autonomy · Non-maleficence · Justice · Dignity · Beneficence

**Hints and Tips:**
- Ethical areas can be very **confusing**
- Speak with a senior doctor in the first instance if you are unsure about a case
- **Read widely** about ethics
- **Debate** and **discuss** ethical areas with your fellow students

*Medical School at a Glance*, First Edition. Rachel K. Thomas © 2017 John Wiley & Sons, Ltd. Published 2017 by John Wiley & Sons, Ltd.

There are **specific principles** that should underlie medicine. While these principles may be clear, they can at times become confusing or **complicated** in daily medical and surgical situations. These principles are included in this chapter to help highlight some areas in your first encounters as a medical student that you should start considering. This is not a detailed exploration of them as ethics is a **dynamic** and **complex area**, and each case requires its own considerations.

There are four main principles, according to the **biomedical ethical framework** (Figure 8.1):

1 Beneficence
2 Non-maleficence
3 Justice
4 Autonomy.

Other important principles include:
• Honesty
• Dignity.

It is important to start **cultivating** these principles when you start at medical school.

There are various **resources** available to help with ethical dilemmas, such as the BMA student ethics toolkit (bma.org.uk/ethics), the Medical Protection Society (www.medicalprotection.org) and the Medical Defence Union (www.themdu.com). The GMC has extensive ethical guidance available online (www.gmc-uk.org).

It can be **difficult** to include all these principles in every interaction but you should use them as a framework to guide your interactions. Remember that every ethical issue you face has its own specific **nuances**, and that at times there are no absolute solutions, only guiding principles.

It is advisable to **read widely** on ethics, and to try to participate in **debates** and **discussions** whenever possible. These can provide useful ways to help learn and practice ethics.

## Beneficence

**Beneficence**, with regards to medical ethics, means doing what is in the **best interest** of the patient. This can be a difficult and complicated area, as at times it may be in the patient's best interests to cease active treatments. This can feel contrary to what you feel the role of a doctor should be.

This area is also complicated when a patient and their doctor have different views on what their 'best interests' are. Ensure that you know the wishes of each patient, particularly with regards to situations such as **advanced directives** and **Do Not Attempt Resuscitation** (DNAR) orders. **End-of-life care** can be confusing and confronting. Teams of members involved in the patient's care usually meet to agree on a consensus and patient's wishes should be respected, unless they involve acts that are not legal.

## Non-maleficence

**Non-maleficence** means not doing any harm. It is a key underlying principle that a doctor must '**first do no harm**', or '*primum*

*non nocere*', a quote that is commonly, but falsely, attributed to the Hippocratic Oath.

This area can become difficult when, for instance, a side effect of a medication, or a risk of a procedure, is so significant as to possibly outweigh the impact of the disease on the patient.

## Justice

**Justice**, in the context of medical ethics, means that **similar patients** should be treated in a **similar way**. You should not let prejudice or bias impact on how treatments are distributed. Justice involves the fair distribution of scarce resources – be they clinical resources of equipment or the more personal resources of your time.

This area can become confusing when it relates to healthcare inequalities. For instance, certain geographical areas have fewer financial resources to provide the same healthcare or treatment options as a neighbouring area, or the high cost of treating one patient can impact on the capability to treat others.

## Autonomy

**Autonomy** represents the **patient's right** to have control over their own decisions. It protects the fact that the patient must be allowed to decide what they want, without being pressured by anyone else.

This area becomes complicated in situations where the patient does not have **capacity** and is therefore unable to give **informed consent** (see Chapter 26). It can also be difficult when patients discharge themselves against medical advice.

## Honesty

**Honesty** is a key part of any relationship between doctor and patient. Honesty is also important in the **consent process**, as a patient needs to have confidence that their doctor is honestly telling them all the required information, both for and against the treatment in question (see Chapter 26).

As a doctor, you expect your patient to be honest with you – ensure that you always pay them the same respect.

This area can become confusing at times, such as when a patient has expressed a wish for less than full disclosure on their condition.

## Dignity

**Dignity** relates to the **sense of worth** of an individual, and must underpin all your interactions –not just at medical school. Its presence helps people feel **valued, capable** and more in **control** of a situation – aspects that are key to promote, as being a patient can lead to an erosion of them.

Dignity needs to be **promoted** and **protected** for all patients, both those with and without **capacity**, and should continue both in **life** and **after death**.

# 9 Communication skills and teamwork

**Figure 9.1** Aspects of communication

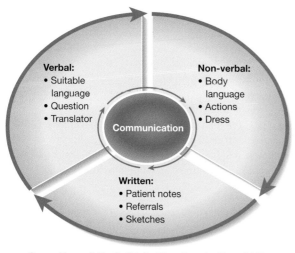

Source: *Thomas R. Practical Medical Procedures at a Glance (2015). Reproduced with permission of John Wiley & Sons Ltd.*

**Figure 9.2** Establishing rapport is important in the doctor-patient relationship

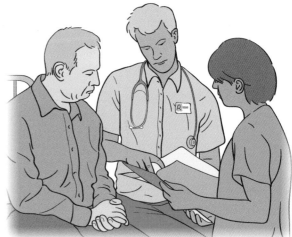

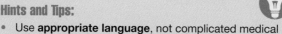

**Hints and Tips:**

- Use **appropriate language**, not complicated medical jargon, when talking with patients
- Remember to use both **verbal** and **non-verbal skills** to build rapport
- Always ask for **help** or **clarification** if required – **never assume anything!**

**Figure 9.3** Good patient care depends upon teamwork

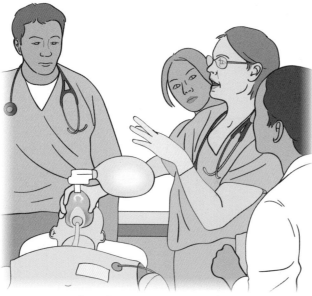

Source: *Thomas R. Practical Medical Procedures at a Glance (2015). Reproduced with permission of John Wiley & Sons Ltd.*

**Situation awareness**

- Anticipation
- Information interpretation
- Questioning
- Work-space modification

**Task management**

- Planning
- Preparing
- Prioritising
- Resource identification and allocation

**Team working**

- Leadership
- Role allocation
- Co-operation
- Communication

**Decision-making**

- Evaluation of risks
- Evaluation of benefits
- Re-evaluation
- Modification

*Medical School at a Glance,* First Edition. Rachel K. Thomas © 2017 John Wiley & Sons, Ltd. Published 2017 by John Wiley & Sons, Ltd.

# Communication skills

**Good communication** is fundamental to being a good clinician, and has many aspects (Figure 9.1). The GMC highlights the importance of effective communication in its document *Good Medical Practice* and there is increasing focus on developing medical students' communication skills by experts in medical education. Clear communication can lead to a better medical interaction, more effective teamwork and, importantly, it also **minimises error** and **improves safety**.

By virtue of having been accepted into medical school, and in many cases having undergone an interview, you are likely to have good communication skills already. However, there is always room for **improvement**. Furthermore, medical interactions often hold **unique challenges,** for instance breaking bad news, which require well-honed communication skills.

## Benefits of good communication

Communication is more than talking. Many people forget that apart from the **verbal** and **non-verbal** elements of communication, it is actually a **two-way process** between **two (or more) parties**. It thus involves both **good listening,** as well as **speaking clearly** and **appropriately** to the party being addressed.

At the doctor–patient interface, good communication can lead to a more comprehensive history and the establishment of a **good rapport** more quickly (Figure 9.2). With rapport and trust, a patient will have a better healthcare experience, often leading to improved **concordance** when it comes to future management plans, and ultimately a **more satisfactory outcome**.

In interactions between medical colleagues, good communication can improve teamwork coordination and improve the transfer of information. This can impact markedly on **patient safety**. One of the most important considerations is to **remember to communicate**. Many medical mistakes occur as a result of failure to **hand over patient information**. Remembering to hand over and communicating **clearly** and **concisely** can significantly minimise error.

## Communicating with patients

**Effective** and **active listening** is the first step for good communication. Be 'present' when the other party speaks – be attentive yet relaxed, and focus on what is being said. When someone starts talking it is easy for thoughts to wander and then find that you have missed part of what the person has said. If this occurs, **ask them to repeat** themselves. You do not want to overlook the one crucial point that could lead to the diagnosis – or miss the patient revealing their severe allergic reaction to penicillin!

Active listening involves **clarifying** with the other party that you understand what they are saying. **Summarise** at convenient intervals and **ask them if there is anything you have omitted.** This not only aids safe information gathering, but also shows the party you have been paying attention to what they have been saying. Such validation can help build rapport.

**Non-verbal** communication is also an important part of communication. Use **open body language** (i.e. avoid crossed arms and angle your body and face towards the other party). **Good eye contact** is reassuring and small affirmative noises can help people feel they are being listened to. **Actions** such as handwashing also aid in building a patient's trust in you.

When you communicate in a medical capacity there are additional things to consider. How you communicate with patients, of course, will vary from patient to patient, with some aspects, such as identification and confidentiality, remaining the same. You should first establish **the patient's understanding** of the situation thus far, and **how much information they would like to know.** It is best to **start simply** and **avoid complicated medical terminology**. **Medical advice leaflets** are commonly available (either physically or online at sites such as www.patient.co.uk). Consider printing a leaflet or suggesting such a site to patients as an adjunct to your conversation. Visiting these sites yourself can also help with your **learning** of common symptoms and treatments for conditions.

## Communicating with healthcare professionals

All of the above tenets of good communication also apply when you are communicating with other medical professionals. When you start formally discussing a patient, your presentation should follow the **standard clerking sequence of history**, **examination, differential diagnosis, investigation results** and **proposed management plan**, as this is the easiest way of communicating all the relevant information. Some clinicians prefer abbreviated versions of the clerking and these are particularly pertinent later in your career when you have to discuss or refer patients over the phone or during emergencies. However, ensure you learn how to use the standard sequence so as to not miss any details while you are learning.

**Practice** is the best way to refine your communication skills and over time, as you complete more interactions and presentations, your expertise will increase. Ask whether you can **accompany doctors** when sensitive communication is required (e.g. breaking bad news). By viewing how they do this, **reflecting** on such situations and then **debriefing** with the team afterwards, you will learn and improve your own communication skills.

## Teamwork

Effective communication contributes to good teamwork, by ensuring the different parties have the same background information and are working together towards an appropriate plan and goal. If you take a moment to analyse the number of professionals who are involved in a single patient's admission, the importance of coordinated teamwork becomes clear. This can most obviously be seen in emergency settings (Figure 9.3).

Being a good team player will stand you in good stead. Aspects of your demeanour and conduct can make a big difference. Being **reliable, punctual, responsible** and **enthusiastic** are invaluable. Colleagues want to work with someone who will **complete jobs** assigned to them and is **personable** as well.

Most of all, **be safe** and if in doubt, **ask.** This is essential to being trusted by your colleagues. Although some people can appear exasperated on being asked questions, asking for clarification is always preferable to endangering the patient.

# 10 Balance

**Figure 10.1** Aspects of life outside of medical school

Hobbies and interests

Religious, spiritual and philosophical concerns

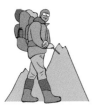
Future plans and projects

Job

Self-care – sport and exercise

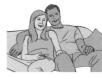
Community activities

Family, relationships

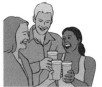
Friends and colleagues

**Figure 10.2** Medical school should be part of a balanced life

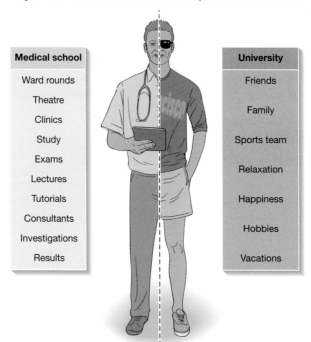

| Medical school | University |
|---|---|
| Ward rounds | Friends |
| Theatre | Family |
| Clinics | Sports team |
| Study | Relaxation |
| Exams | Happiness |
| Lectures | Hobbies |
| Tutorials | Vacations |
| Consultants | |
| Investigations | |
| Results | |

*Medical School at a Glance*, First Edition. Rachel K. Thomas © 2017 John Wiley & Sons, Ltd. Published 2017 by John Wiley & Sons, Ltd.

There is more to life than medicine and it is important to bear that in mind as you progress through your career. Being a medical professional can be an all-consuming job and thus activities and 'downtime' outside of the clinical environment are essential (Figure 10.1). Furthermore, interviewers often look at your **achievements outside of medicine**, to better assess what type of person you are and whether you maintain balance in your life (Figure 10.2).

In addition to the basic requirements of high academic achievement, medical schools tend to select individuals with **all-round capability** and performance. Many people continue the extracurricular activities started in school, possibly those also enjoyed throughout higher education and perhaps beyond. If you find yourself letting your prior activities go, not to worry, university is an excellent place to begin new interests or to rekindle older ones. Most universities hold **freshers' fairs** where you can find out about numerous university societies. Medical schools also often have their own **clubs** and a **committee** that organises events and welfare for medical students.

Joining a '**MedSoc**'(or any other) **committee** is also a good idea if it appeals to you. Being elected to a role and then engaging in committee meetings is not only a **highly social** (and hopefully fun) activity, but you can learn important leadership, organisational and teamwork skills too.

You may wish to look outside the university setting for additional inspiration. A quick **online search** will reveal many activities and clubs in your town. By joining **mailing lists** you can be pointed in the direction of upcoming interesting events. **Volunteering** also appeals to many people and your library should be able to provide you with further information on local charities.

If you feel you would like to attend additional medically orientated activities, the **Royal Society of Medicine** is an excellent place to start, as it has a web page dedicated to advertising its events.

Make sure you **keep certificates** of any events or courses that you attend as you can include these in your **portfolio** later on, as proof of attendance.

## Fitting extracurricular activities into your time

Regardless of the activities you choose to pursue, having a **scheduled commitment** outside of medicine will mean you have designated leisure time each week, which you are less likely to sacrifice. **Good time management**, which is a skill that you will develop, allows you to fit medical studies as well as your extracurricular activities into the working week, even when you have exams. **Keeping a diary** or **making a plan** of the upcoming week and scheduling commitments, meetings and study sessions will make your life easier.

Many people prefer more **flexible leisure activities** that do not necessarily require formal attendance (e.g. reading or cooking). If that is the case, it is still advisable to ensure you plan these activities into your schedule. Otherwise they can be taken over by other work pursuits such as study. Of course, there may be times when you have to forgo your usual leisure activities for an unexpected work-related issue. However, you should try to avoid this becoming a habit.

It is especially important to continue to make time for **relaxation** around exams. **Exercise,** be that team sports, going to the gym or something as simple as a walk outdoors, is **particularly beneficial** to **physical** and **mental health.** Adjusting your schedule to allow for additional study at exam time may be required, but try not to sacrifice all your leisure time. You will find that after a leisure pursuit you are likely to be refreshed, and can actually study better and remember more.

## Keeping perspective

It is all too easy to get bogged down in the medical life. This is especially true during the medical student years when there is an almost continuous obstacle course of exams and assessments. If you find yourself struggling with medicine, it is worthwhile taking a moment to reflect. **Leisure activities, time with family and friends, regular meals** and a **good night's sleep** will often make the weariest of us feel restored and more focused.

Often, going back to basics and reminding yourself of why you pursued a career in medicine in the first place can help you regain perspective. Look back on past **medical school personal statements** to remember your original reasons for applying. **Make a list of pros and cons** of medicine. More than likely, you will find more pros than cons. Try to **reflect on good experiences** and **things that you have done well**. Keeping a **real-time list** will help and you can look back on it for inspiration and motivation.

If you still find yourself struggling, remember there are a wealth of sources of help (see Chapter 6), and even alternate paths you can follow if you find yourself continuing to doubt if a career in medicine is for you (see Chapter 36).

**Hints and Tips:**
- Ask for **help early**
- **Schedule leisure activities** – and stick to the schedule whenever possible
- Ensure that you eat, exercise and sleep **regularly**, especially during exam time. You cannot perform optimally if you do not **look after yourself**

# 11 Evidence-based medicine

**Figure 11.1** Components of evidence-based medicine (EBM)

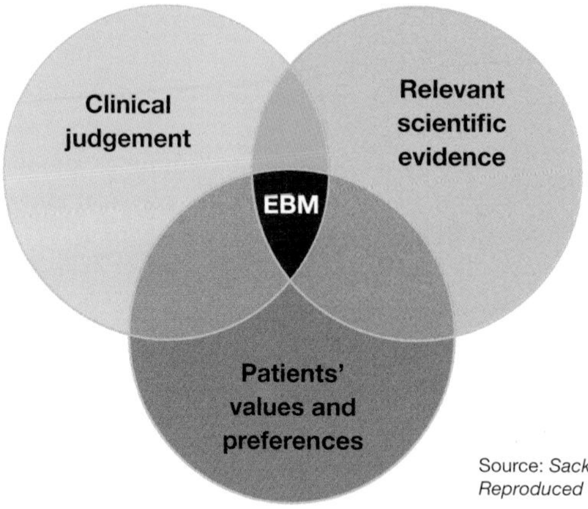

Clinical judgement

Relevant scientific evidence

EBM

Patients' values and preferences

Source: *Sackett DL et al. BMJ 1996; 312 (7023): 71-72. Reproduced with permission of BMJ Publishing Ltd.*

**Figure 11.2** Stages in a clinical audit

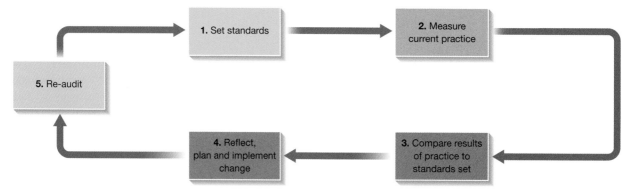

1. Set standards

2. Measure current practice

5. Re-audit

4. Reflect, plan and implement change

3. Compare results of practice to standards set

**Figure 11.3** EBM evidence pyramid

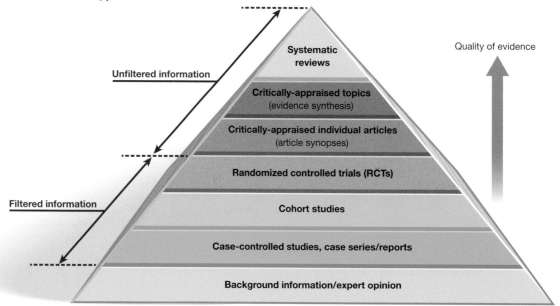

Unfiltered information

Filtered information

Quality of evidence

Systematic reviews

Critically-appraised topics (evidence synthesis)

Critically-appraised individual articles (article synopses)

Randomized controlled trials (RCTs)

Cohort studies

Case-controlled studies, case series/reports

Background information/expert opinion

Source: *EBM Pyramid and EBM Page Generator. © 2006 Trustees of Dartmouth College and Yale University. All Rights Reserved. Produced by Jan Glover, David Izzo, Karen Odato and Lei Wang.*

Evidence-based medicine (EBM) has enabled a more **critical, systematic** and **scientific approach** to clinical practice than was employed previously. It involves a process of systematically reviewing, appraising and implementing clinical research findings to help deliver **optimum clinical care** to patients (Figure 11.1).

It has turned clinical medicine from using traditional, anecdotal and theoretical reasoning based on basic science, to using real data and evidence from high quality **randomised controlled trials** and **observational studies.** This is also combined with the patient's needs and wishes, and with clinical expertise. Overall, EBM has made clinical practice more empirically and scientifically grounded, helping to achieve more consistent, safer and cost-effective clinical care.

EBM is included in medical school curricula to differing degrees. It is present in many **clinical guidelines** and **protocols** for **best practice** and, as a student, these can be very helpful in learning how to **manage** diseases. As a medical student, EBM can also be used in **research** and **audits.** However, as EBM is constantly evolving and improving, it can lead to challenges in staying up-to-date.

## Clinical audits

**Clinical audits** are a systematic way of **assessing, evaluating** and **improving** patient care (Figure 11.2). According to the GMC, doctors should take part in **regular audits.** These audits involve various stages which depend upon the audit itself, but include determining best practice (which EBM can be used for), measuring how often this is the case, taking action or developing a framework to improve how often this is the case, and then monitoring to ensure that the improvements are sustained.

## The clinical question

In EBM, a **well-defined clinical question** is key. A popular method to formulate a clinical question on an intervention is based on the **PICO** format where:

**P** *Patient/population/participants* you are interested in. Is there an age group, gender or population?
**I** *Intervention*. What is the management strategy you are looking for? Is it a diagnostic test (e.g. value of MRI) or exposure (e.g. use of a chemotherapy agent) that is of interest?
**C** *Comparator*. What is your control group? Is there a control group? What is the 'alternative management strategy?'
**O** *Outcome*. What is your measured clinical outcome/patient related consequences of the intervention. This outcome could be the length of hospital stay, mortality or improvement in a clinical marker (e.g. inflammatory markers).

For example, looking at the impact of handwashing on the neonatal ward, P = the babies admitted to the neonatal unit, I = handwashing by all the visitors to the neonatal unit, C = no handwashing by all the visitors to the neonatal unit, O = number of infections in the neonates admitted to the ward. Useful things to add are the time period you are interested in (e.g. number of visitors per day measured for 1 week and number of neonatal infections over the following 2 weeks).

Although the most common type of EBM questions are based on **interventions** or **diagnostic tests**, alternative types of EBM questions include questions about **aetiology, diagnosis** or **prognosis**. In these cases, although the whole PICO format cannot be used, thinking about the PICO can still help to focus the search and to formulate a suitable question.

## Reviewing the literature and reading papers

The basis of EBM is a **literature review**, which is a search for all the studies published related to your clinical question.

Your university library may run courses on performing a literature review that you could attend, or else you could follow tutorials published online by the **Cochrane Collaboration**.

Reading a scientific paper is a **skill** – one that is commonly tested in written examinations. When reading the paper, it can help to think about their 'PICO'.

Every study, particularly interventional studies, can be classified into observational or randomised controlled trials (RCTs). The hierarchy of evidence from the literature is pyramid shaped with **systematic reviews** at the top (Figure 11.3). The **hierarchy of evidence** can also be categorised into grades where **Grade A**, based on **Level 1a evidence,** is the **highest** (a systematic review based on high quality RCTs and meta-analysis) and **Grade D**, based on **Level 5 evidence**, is the lowest (expert opinion).

A systematic review is an overview of primary studies that contains:
- Objectives
- Sources
- Methods

and is:
- Explicit
- Transparent
- Reproducible.

The **most reliable systematic reviews** are notably those undertaken by the **Cochrane Collaboration,** because they **regularly update** and review the evidence. The Cochrane Collaboration also has guidelines available on how to perform a systematic review and what makes a good systematic review. A systematic review is 'above' (stronger evidence than) an RCT because it looks at all the RCTs in that study, thereby reducing the risk of any bias from an individual study.

**Systematic bias** is when comparisons are distorted, or there are erroneous influences on the conclusions about the groups involved. Having a high level of bias means that you cannot trust whether the results are due to the intervention or something else. Different study designs require different steps to reduce bias. RCTs theoretically avoid bias by selecting a sample of participants and allocating them randomly to the different groups. However, bias can still occur in RCTs.

## General advice

There is a lot to learn about EBM. It can seem daunting at first, particularly if you do not have a statistics background. Try to continue to develop your knowledge in this topic by reading papers, participating in journal clubs and reading about EBM while at medical school. A good understanding of EBM is key to understanding **current medical practice** as a **competent doctor**.

Before embarking on a literature review or reading a scientific paper ensure that you understand the topic and the intervention. If the clinical condition is completely new to you, a clinical review in a high-impact journal can give you a summary of the topic.

**Hints and Tips**
- The more papers you read on a topic, the better you will become at reading papers and the more you will understand the topic itself.

# 12 Understanding guidelines

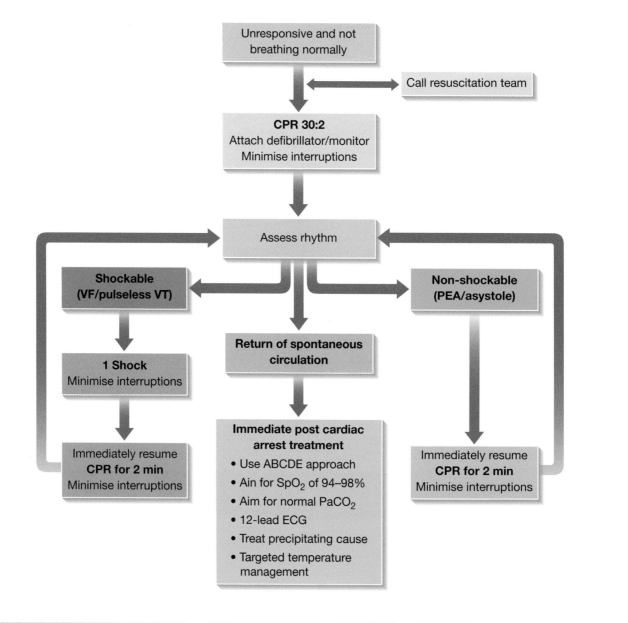

**Figure 12.1**  Adult advanced life support algorithm

Unresponsive and not breathing normally

Call resuscitation team

**CPR 30:2**
Attach defibrillator/monitor
Minimise interruptions

Assess rhythm

**Shockable
(VF/pulseless VT)**

**Non-shockable
(PEA/asystole)**

**1 Shock**
Minimise interruptions

**Return of spontaneous
circulation**

Immediately resume
**CPR for 2 min**
Minimise interruptions

**Immediate post cardiac
arrest treatment**
• Use ABCDE approach
• Ain for SpO$_2$ of 94–98%
• Aim for normal PaCO$_2$
• 12-lead ECG
• Treat precipitating cause
• Targeted temperature
management

Immediately resume
**CPR for 2 min**
Minimise interruptions

**During CPR**
• Ensure high quality chest compressions
• Minimise interruptions to compressions
• Give oxygen
• Use waveform capnography
• Continuous compressions when advanced airway in place
• Vascular access (intravenous or intraosseous)
• Give adrenaline every 3–5 min
• Give amiodarone after 3 shocks

**Treat reversible causes**
• Hypoxia
• Hypovolaemia
• Hypo-/hyperkalaemia/metabolic
• Hypothemia
• Thrombosis – coronary or pulmonary
• Tension pneumothorax
• Tamponade – cardiac
• Toxins

**Consider**
• Ultrasound imaging
• Mechanical chest compressions to facilitate transfer/treatment
• Coronary angiography and percutaneous coronary intervention
• Extracorporeal CPR

Source: *Adult Life Support (2015). Reproduced with permission of Resuscitation Council (UK). (https://www.resus.org.uk/resuscitation-guidelines/)*

*Medical School at a Glance*, First Edition. Rachel K. Thomas © 2017 John Wiley & Sons, Ltd. Published 2017 by John Wiley & Sons, Ltd.

Medicine has moved away from the 'maverick doctor' and shifted towards **evidence-based medicine** (see Chapter 11). This has been shown to be better for **patient care** and greatly helps you as a junior doctor to manage a patient safely. This chapter provides a brief introduction to guidelines and protocols and gives resources on where to access these. **Guidelines** are a valuable learning tool, as they are updated more frequently than textbooks and can indicate current hospital management plans.

Guidelines are **recommendations** issued by large organisations on how to manage common medical problems or conditions. Guidelines are very useful tools; however, they are recommendations on how to manage and investigate patients, not absolute rules. There may be several different guidelines on the same topics. Most of the time guidelines will be followed, but at times, under the guidance of senior input at the hospital, they are not. If you encounter a situation where the guidelines have not been followed, try to understand why the guidance was not followed, **reflect** on this, and speak to a senior doctor to help understand why this was the case.

## Types of guidelines

Every hospital also has its own guidelines, called **local guidelines**. These are often based on **national guidelines;** however, they might vary depending on, for example, the resources available to that local population. Certain guidelines, such as **antimicrobial policy**, change depending on the Trust because of the **commonly encountered strains** of bacteria and **local resistance patterns**. It is important when you change hospital that you manage patients in accordance with the relevant local guidelines. Therefore, it is key to research the commonly used guidelines of that area, and understand them, on each clinical placement, both in medical school and in your future career.

During medical school, if you are unable to find national or local guidelines related to a particular topic, look at guidelines from other reputable international, national or hospital sources such as the European Society of Cardiology, the Mayo Clinic in the USA or The Royal Children's Hospital, Melbourne, in Australia. PubMed online is a reliable resource for researching guidelines. These are not always be relevant to practice in the UK but provide reliable summaries of the evidence which can help with your learning.

## Sources of guidelines

Guidelines are published by a variety of **sources**. These include international and national organisations and also the **Royal Colleges**. Every medical specialty has its own Royal College and often these Colleges will endorse guidelines specific to the management of particular medical conditions.

Common sources include the following.

**International guidance**

- World Health Organization (WHO): http://www.who.int/publications/guidelines/en/

**National guidance**

- Resuscitation Council: www.resus.org.uk (useful for algorithms on how to manage the acutely unwell patient; Figure 12.1)
- National Institute for Health and Care Excellence (NICE): https://www.nice.org.uk/guidance (general guidelines for commonly encountered medical disorders, the use of new medical and surgical therapies)
- General Medical Council: www.gmc-uk.org/guidance/good_medical_practice.asp (should be read by every doctor entering clinical practice in the UK)
- National Clinical Guideline Centre: www.ncgc.ac.uk/Guidelines/Our-Publications/ (assimilation of NICE, Royal College of Physicians, Royal College of General Practitioners and Royal College of Nursing guidelines sponsored by the Department of Health)
- Scottish Intercollegiate Guidelines Institute: www.sign.ac.uk (Scottish version of NICE, often has a few additional guidelines to NICE)
- British Thoracic Society: www.brit-thoracic.org.uk (useful for guidelines on common respiratory conditions like chronic obstructive pulmonary disease, asthma, pneumonia)
- Green Book: https://www.gov.uk/government/collections/immunisation-against-infectious-disease-the-green-book (useful for the administration of immunisations)
- Driver and Vehicle Licensing Agency (DVLA): https://www.gov.uk/guidance/current-medical-guidelines-dvla-guidance-for-professionals (for patients with medical conditions who drive)

**Medical colleges**

- Royal College of Physicians: https://www.rcplondon.ac.uk/guidelines-policy
- Royal College of Surgeons: https://www.rcseng.ac.uk/fds/publications-clinical-guidelines/clinical_guidelines/index.html (some of the guidelines relate to dentistry)
- Royal College of Obstetricians and Gynaecologists: https://www.rcog.org.uk/guidelines (their green top guidelines are very useful for learning about common O&G emergencies)
- Royal College of General Practitioners (via the national clinical guidelines centre): http://www.rcgp.org.uk/clinical-and-research/clinical-resources/national-clinical-guideline-centre.aspx
- Royal College of Paediatrics and Child Health: http://www.rcpch.ac.uk/improving-child-health/clinical-guidelines-and-standards/published-rcpch/clinical-guidelines-and-sta
- Royal College of Psychiatrists: http://www.rcpsych.ac.uk/usefulresources/publications.aspx

**Hints and Tips:**

When reading a guideline, try to take into account:
- **When** it was published
- **Who** published it (national guidelines or a group of experts in the field)
- **Who** the target audience is

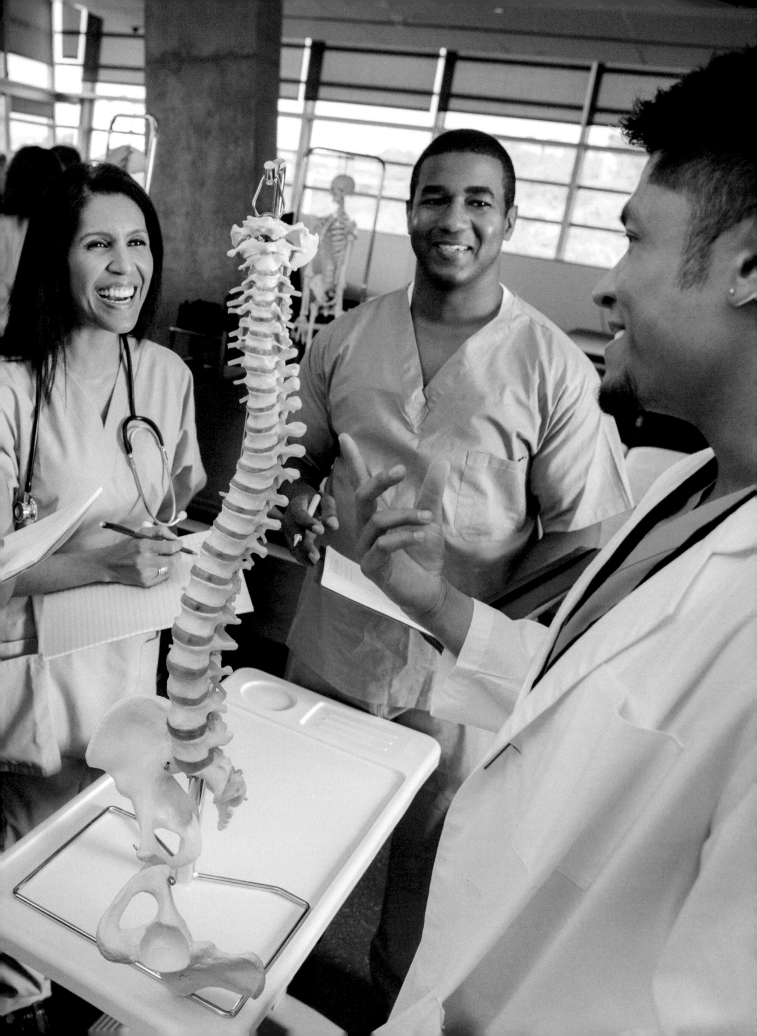

# Starting clinical activities

Part 3

## Chapters

## 13 Behaving on the ward

**Figure 13.1** Appropriate ward attire

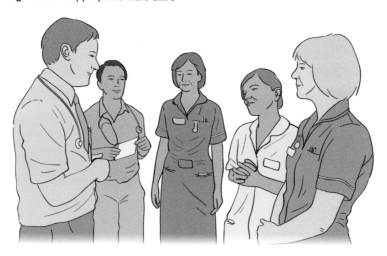

**Figure 13.2** Correlating theoretical and clinical knowledge

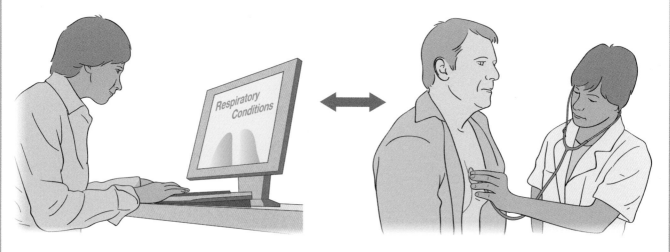

**Figure 13.3** Some hospitals clearly show where drug rounds are occurring

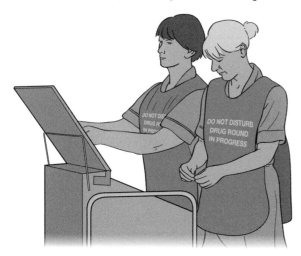

**Hints and Tips:**
- **Introduce yourself** to the nursing staff present on the ward
- If appropriate, ask the staff if there might be any **suitable patients** you could speak with or examine – the staff will know the patients best
- If you are unsure of ward behaviour, **ask** a member of staff

*Medical School at a Glance*, First Edition. Rachel K. Thomas © 2017 John Wiley & Sons, Ltd. Published 2017 by John Wiley & Sons, Ltd.

## Suitable general behaviour on the ward

**Ward-based activities** are a **mainstay** of **clinical care**. There are **different types** of wards, and each can require **different behaviour at times,** but there are **general rules** dictating appropriate overall behaviour.

Always behave **politely** and **courteously** to all **patients,** and **colleagues.** Remember that you are training to be a **medical professional,** and that you are thus representing medical professionals each time you are on the ward, even while you are still a student. Do not make inappropriate jokes, use inappropriate language or behave in a discourteous manner – and do not abscond from the wards thinking no-one will notice, as they will! And you will miss out on **key learning opportunities.**

As with any clinical interaction, basic steps such as **handwashing** must be performed (see Chapter 7). It is preferable to perform this in **full view** of the patient, so that they can be reassured that it has occurred. Ensure that you respect **patient confidentiality,** taking care to only discuss patients in appropriately separate areas and at appropriate volumes (see Chapter 7). **Draw curtains closed** around the bed, particularly when examining a patient, to assist with privacy, but remember that curtains are not sound proof! Some wards, such as paediatric wards, encourage a more relaxed interaction with patients, to help the children to feel more comfortable.

Your behaviour will greatly impact on your experiences on the ward. If you are **polite, friendly** and **helpful** to nursing staff, they will be more approachable. Ensure that you **introduce** yourself to them, and ensure that you do **not interfere** with clinical commitments. For instance, it is inappropriate to interact and distract patients at **meal times,** and in most Healthcare Trusts these times are 'protected'. Similarly, it is important not to interrupt staff on **medication rounds** (Figure 13.3). The care of the patient is the primary concern, and while your learning is important, it is secondary to this.

## Suitable attire on the ward

Most clinical scenarios have clearly prescribed clothing regulations. If these are not explicitly stipulated, the default should be **neat professional attire.** Many Healthcare Trusts have a 'bare below the elbows' policy. This means that no item of clothing should extend to cover the lower arm (Figure 13.1). Clothing that does extend below the elbow interferes with thorough **handwashing,** leading to inadequate hygiene and a greater risk of infection transmission (see Chapter 7). It can be helpful to carry around a small container of **gel** or **alcohol-based hand rub** (ABHR) to clean your hands with. If **ties** are worn, they are best tucked in – loose, flapping ties can pose an infection risk.

Ensure that medical school or Healthcare Trust **identification badges** are worn and visible at all times.

**Surgical wards** may permit the wearing of **surgical scrubs,** but this is dependent upon local protocols. Some Healthcare Trusts aim to minimise their use outside of theatre, and many prohibit them being worn in public eating areas.

Footwear should be **neat, clean** and **professional.** If scrubs are worn, more casual shoes may be permitted. Generally, **theatre shoes** should be reserved for use in theatre only (see Chapter 14).

## Learning on the ward

**Ward-based learning** is a **crucially important** way of gaining **clinical skills.** It is advisable to become **comfortable** with patients and with being on the ward early on in your training. It is normal to experience a few nerves when placed in a **new environment** – increasing your exposure to these new environments will naturally help make you feel more confident and more comfortable, which will, in turn, enable you to **focus** more fully on the patient and on your learning.

**Taking histories** (see Chapter 19) and **performing clinical examinations** (see Chapter 20) need to be practised extensively. After gaining an understanding of these by practising on your fellow students, friends or family members, seeing patients will greatly increase your skills and knowledge. Many students find it helpful to closely correlate the gaining of **clinical knowledge** with **theoretical knowledge,** as one helps the other. It is advisable to **read** about a condition before **seeing** a patient with that condition. Then **re-reading** about the condition, after having **discussed** aspects of it with the patient and colleagues, can help to cement the condition in your mind (Figure 13.2).

Try to determine **how** you learn best – by seeing, hearing or interacting (see Chapter 4). If you are unsure of your most efficient **learning modality,** ensure that you cover material in different ways. Explaining concepts and presenting to fellow students can be good ways to maximise learning.

Many patients are happy for students to spend time with them. Remember that patients are in hospital for their own reasons, and if one is kind enough to permit you to spend time with them, be appropriately **appreciative** and **respectful.**

Respect any **limitations** that the patient has, and **moderate** the time you spend with them according to their capabilities. For instance, if a patient is very short of breath, respect this limitation when trying to take their history.

When with a patient, be sure to ask for help early if you have concerns about the **patient's condition deteriorating** (see Chapter 18). Do not provide clinical information unless permitted to do so, and if a patient has any questions, be sure to pass these on to a qualified colleague.

Pay attention to **confidentiality** when you are learning from a patient. If you discuss a patient with other members of your team or fellow students, ensure that you do so discreetly. General discussions to help your learning, focusing on management, worst-case scenarios and prognosis may be irrelevant for the patient at hand – but very confusing or concerning if overheard, as they may naturally assume that they are the ones who are being discussed. Ensure that any notes you take are disposed of in a **confidential waste bin** or shredded.

**Ward rounds** can be very busy, but can also be excellent learning opportunities. Try to help the junior doctors by, for instance, helping to collect patient notes. **Shadowing** junior doctors can also be very beneficial, especially for an understanding of day-to-day tasks and important activities such as **discharge planning** (see Chapter 30).

# 14 Behaving in theatre

**Figure 14.1** Scrubs

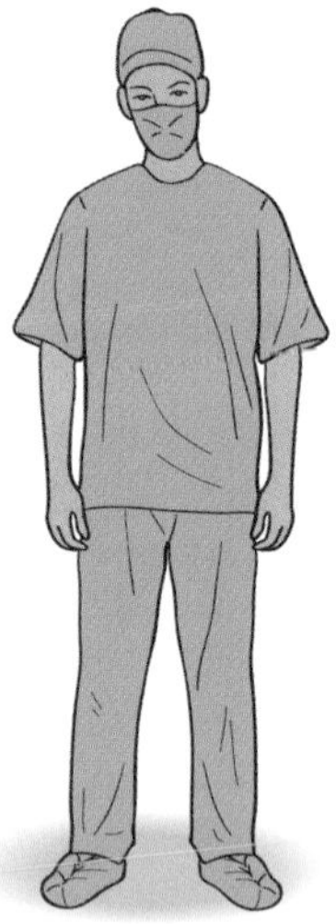

**Figure 14.2** Scrubbing in

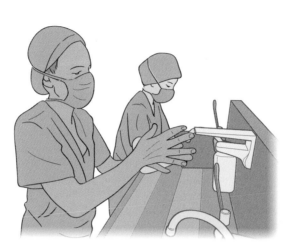

**Figure 14.3** How to move around the theatre

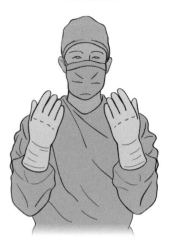

**Figure 14.4** WHO surgical checklist

## Surgical Safety Checklist

World Health Organization | Patient Safety
A World Alliance for Safer Health Care

### Before induction of anaesthesia

(with at least nurse and anaesthetist)

**Has the patient confirmed his/her identity, site, procedure, and consent?**
- ☐ Yes

**Is the site marked?**
- ☐ Yes
- ☐ Not applicable

**Is the anaesthesia machine and medication check complete?**
- ☐ Yes

**Is the pulse oximeter on the patient and functioning?**
- ☐ Yes

**Does the patient have a:**

**Known allergy?**
- ☐ No
- ☐ Yes

**Difficult airway or aspiration risk?**
- ☐ No
- ☐ Yes, and equipment/assistance available

**Risk of >500ml blood loss (7ml/kg in children)?**
- ☐ No
- ☐ Yes, and two IVs/central access and fluids planned

### Before skin incision

(with nurse, anaesthetist and surgeon)

- ☐ Confirm all team members have introduced themselves by name and role.
- ☐ Confirm the patient's name, procedure, and where the incision will be made.

**Has antibiotic prophylaxis been given within the last 60 minutes?**
- ☐ Yes
- ☐ Not applicable

**Anticipated Critical Events**

**To Surgeon:**
- ☐ What are the critical or non-routine steps?
- ☐ How long will the case take?
- ☐ What is the anticipated blood loss?

**To Anaesthetist:**
- ☐ Are there any patient-specific concerns?

**To Nursing Team:**
- ☐ Has sterility (including indicator results) been confirmed?
- ☐ Are there equipment issues or any concerns?

**Is essential imaging displayed?**
- ☐ Yes
- ☐ Not applicable

### Before patient leaves operating room

(with nurse, anaesthetist and surgeon)

**Nurse Verbally Confirms:**
- ☐ The name of the procedure
- ☐ Completion of instrument, sponge and needle counts
- ☐ Specimen labelling (read specimen labels aloud, including patient name)
- ☐ Whether there are any equipment problems to be addressed

**To Surgeon, Anaesthetist and Nurse:**
- ☐ What are the key concerns for recovery and management of this patient?

This checklist is not intended to be comprehensive. Additions and modifications to fit local practice are encouraged.          Revised 1 / 2009          © WHO, 2009

Source: *Reproduced with permission of WHO, 2009.*

**Hints and Tips:**
- **Introduce yourself** to the team
- Be mindful and maintain **infection control procedures**
- **Read** about the **procedure** beforehand
- **Read** about the **case** beforehand and **later reflect** on the case

*Medical School at a Glance*, First Edition. Rachel K. Thomas © 2017 John Wiley & Sons, Ltd. Published 2017 by John Wiley & Sons, Ltd.

# The theatre

Theatre is where patients have **surgeries** or **'sterile procedures'**. The reason there is a separate room to perform these procedures is because all the equipment is available in one place, both for the surgical and anaesthetic teams and for infection control reasons. Theatres are built with **special ventilation systems** and other **infection control measures** to minimise the risk of infection. This means that theatre is often a very well-run, well-regulated environment where you will have to observe certain 'rules'.

Initially, you may feel in the way and out of place as a medical student in **theatre**, or the **operating room (OR)**. This should not discourage you, as being in theatre is an excellent **learning experience** and this chapter aims to give you some basic advice on how to maximise your learning in this environment.

## General 'rules' for theatre

Ensure that you are familiar with the **local protocols** for the theatre you are attending, as these can differ.

Make sure you know which team you are shadowing or attached to. **Introduce** yourself to that team. Introduce yourself to the **nurse in charge** of the theatre, explain why you are there and which team you are linked with.

As part of **infection control**, you will have to change into **scrubs**, wear a hair cap, remove any jewellery and, potentially, change into special theatre shoes (which are often Crocs® or clogs; Figure 14.1). You cannot carry bags with you into theatre and will have to leave them in the changing room. If you anticipate that you will be in theatre do not bring valuables. Nails should be short, earrings should be studs without stones and hair should be tied back. You will also be expected to enter theatre from a **specific door**, which is usually separate from where the patient will be anaesthetised. Finding the change room, the scrubs (which are usually in the change room) and the correct theatre once you are dressed can all take a while, so ensure that you leave plenty of **time. Never enter the induction room while the anaesthetist is putting the patient to sleep.** This can cause complications for the patient.

**Aseptic procedures** are carried out in theatres. Maintaining a **sterile field** in the operating theatre is key to minimise the risks of infection. The operating team, who are in direct contact with the patient, are **scrubbed up** (scrubbed in). This means that they wash their hands very thoroughly and change into special gowns, face masks and gloves that are **sterile** (clean and hypothetically free from bacteria; Figure 14.2). To remain 'sterile' the person scrubbed up can only touch other things that are sterile. If they touch something that is not sterile they have to change their gowns and gloves and scrub up again. As a medical student, scrubbing up is a useful thing to learn and will also potentially allow you to be able to observe procedures from a closer angle. If you are **not scrubbed up**, be mindful that the operating team are and try not to touch them, as if you do you will contaminate them. If you **are scrubbed up**, make sure you know where your hands are at all times, and move carefully around the theatre (Figure 14.3). If your glasses or face mask need adjusting, ask someone who is not scrubbed up to adjust them for you, as doing so yourself will contaminate your hands.

Theatre is often a cold environment. However, if you are scrubbed up it can get warm, and some operations mean you will be standing for prolonged periods of time (e.g. 3–4 hours). If you start to feel **faint**, excuse yourself and try to leave the vicinity of the patient. Sit down on the nearest stool and compose yourself. Tell the scrub nurse you are feeling unwell, de-scrub and then leave the theatre to get a drink. You may be able to come back later to observe. To try to prevent this from happening, make sure you are **well-hydrated** beforehand and do some **exercise** (e.g. standing on your tiptoes) to reduce venous pooling of blood in the legs.

Remember that even though the patient is asleep, ensure you maintain **confidentiality** at all times.

## Theatre learning opportunities

**Shadowing surgical teams** enables you to learn about **common procedures** performed in various specialties in theatre, (e.g. laparoscopic cholecystectomy, appendectomy, caesarean section). To maximise your learning, try to **read** about the **procedure** beforehand. Also try to follow the 'patient's journey' from entry through the hospital door to the recovery room. This will give you a better understanding of how the **patient feels**, how the **teams interact** and how to **manage common surgical pre- or postoperative problems**.

Some medical schools offer an **anaesthetic placement**. For a medical student this means learning about the application of basic science to clinical care and proactive thinking (preparing for complications, e.g. pain, blood loss, accessing a difficult airway or intravenous access). It is also a great practical learning experience.

Theatres are also a good place to learn your **practical procedures** (see Chapter 16). Common theatre learning opportunities include catheterisation, cannulation, how to scrub up, aseptic preparation of the patient and how to gain IV access.

## Theatre protocols

The **WHO safety checklist** is a **nationally used guideline** to improve the safety of patients underdoing surgery (Figure 14.4). It is a checklist to ensure that all conditions are optimal for **patient safety**. There are three separate sections:

1 Before induction of anaesthesia
2 Before incision to the skin
3 Before the patient leaves theatre.

Common things that are included are ensuring that it is the correct patient, that consent has been given, any allergies have been identified, the surgical site, everyone in the room has been introduced (name and role) and instrument checks are carried out.

Other **theatre protocols** are **hospital specific**. It is useful to read these before attending theatre. These include scrubbing and gowning, handwashing, airway management and postoperative pain relief. Always ensure that you are familiar with the local protocols, and if in doubt, ask.

**Behaving in clinic**

**Figure 15.1** Possible layouts for a consultation

Patient

Doctor

Student

**'Sitting in' as observer**

Patient

Doctor

Student

**Three way consultation**

Patient

Doctor

Student

**'Hot seating'**

**Figure 15.2** Acting as a chaperone in a clinic

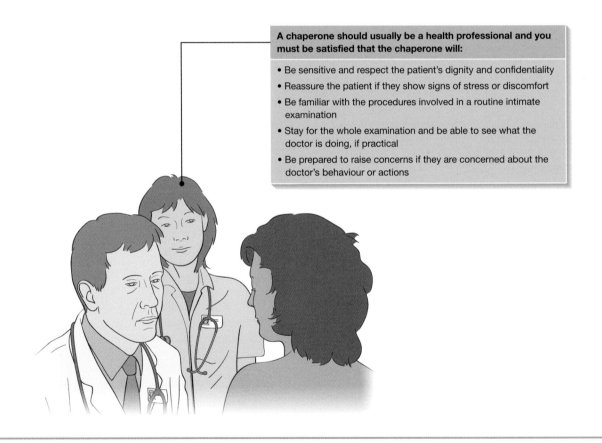

**A chaperone should usually be a health professional and you must be satisfied that the chaperone will:**

- Be sensitive and respect the patient's dignity and confidentiality
- Reassure the patient if they show signs of stress or discomfort
- Be familiar with the procedures involved in a routine intimate examination
- Stay for the whole examination and be able to see what the doctor is doing, if practical
- Be prepared to raise concerns if they are concerned about the doctor's behaviour or actions

*Medical School at a Glance,* First Edition. Rachel K. Thomas © 2017 John Wiley & Sons, Ltd. Published 2017 by John Wiley & Sons, Ltd.

# Outpatient clinic

Outpatient clinics are **pre-arranged appointments** where outpatients attend during a specific time slot, in order to see a doctor. They may see a **Consultant**, their Specialist Registrar, or occasionally more junior members of the team who are more fully supervised. The structure and layout of clinics **vary enormously**, depending on the Trust, hospital, department and specialty, and doctor in charge.

Usually, patients are sent a letter to **attend** the clinic for several reasons:
- Referral from primary care (GP)
- Referral from other secondary care (another specialty)
- Multi-disciplinary input (e.g. Oncology)
- Multi-professional input (e.g. diabetes)
- Diagnosis and formulation of a management plan
- Follow-up after treatment or observation.

Clinics are run to **timetables** specified well in advance, and so you should take the initiative to attend clinics to aid your learning. Find out the timing of particular clinics, and ask other students about which clinics are helpful to attend.

Clinics are an interface between **primary** and **secondary care**, and are an important avenue for learning. Clinics offer the opportunity to learn about the **continuity of care** in a way that many other environments do not. They are largely underused for teaching. Always remember that the patient's clinical care comes before your learning, although the two do not have to be mutually exclusive.

Some hospitals also have **walk-in clinics** or **ambulatory care clinics**.

# Behaving in clinic

As with any clinical encounter, ensure that you are dressed appropriately and **respectfully** when attending a clinic (see Chapter 13). Consider the room layout to help facilitate your learning and to maximise patient comfort (Figure 15.1).

Ensure that you maintain an **attentive** and interested posture, and do not yawn or eat during the clinic.

While you are there to learn, you may also be able to **help** the running of the clinic. It can be helpful to offer to call the patients for your senior, or to help with collecting or opening the patient notes. (This can be particularly helpful if paper notes are used). Some clinicians let you take and present a part of the patient's history, if the patient consents and time permits. Many clinics are run to a **tight schedule**, and so ensure that you are not delaying the clinic for your own educational reasons.

Always **introduce yourself** to the doctors and nurses running the clinic, and to each patient as they enter (although usually the doctor in charge will do this). Ensure that the patient is happy for you to sit in on their consultation by seeking their **consent** (see Chapter 26). If a patient would prefer your were not in the room, do not feel offended, simply **wait outside** the clinic room, use the time to learn something else and enter the room again when the patient leaves.

It is preferable to stay for the **duration** of the clinic, rather than sitting in on a couple of patients, although this will vary depending on the doctor who is running the clinic.

# Learning in clinic

Clinics are an effective place to learn, but this learning is **opportunistic**. The clinic consultations usually last longer than the time spent with patients on ward rounds, and while clinics can be very busy, there is usually enough time to ask questions of your senior either between cases or at the end of the clinic.

Prior to a patient entering the examination room, try to skim their **notes**, or at the very least their **referral letter**, so that you have an idea of why they are in the clinic.

If the hospital has **electronic patient records,** and you have permission to access them, it is very beneficial to learning to take the time to go through these notes and clinic reviews.

Learning in clinics can be assisted if you **create objectives** for what you plan to cover. Setting clear goals can help you determine your learning objectives, and then help you to realise what you have successfully learned – a great morale booster.

Clinics are useful for teaching **communication skills**, and giving a fuller understanding of the impact of disease in the '**real world**'.

Ensure that you also spend time with different teams within the clinic, such as **specialist nurses**, if possible.

Remember that a patient may **consent** to have you in the consultation room while they are speaking with the doctors, but may not wish to have you present for their examination, so ensure that you gain **consent** for this also. Depending on local guidelines, in some cases you may be able to help by acting as a **chaperone**, if the patient requests one (Figure 15.2). A chaperone is a **witness** for the examination, who acts as a **safeguard** for both the medical practitioner and the patient, and is usually another **healthcare professional**. If a chaperone is used, or you act in this capacity, it needs to be documented. If you are seeing a patient yourself, remember to offer them a chaperone, who could potentially be someone else from the team, such as a nurse or doctor.

Subject to the patient's permission, clinics can be a good place to **elicit abnormal signs** and see pathology.

**Reflect** upon your learning at the end of the clinic, assessing how well you have met your goals. **Reflection** can also help guide you towards suitable **additional theoretical follow-up reading**.

**Hints and Tips:**
- Ask to **attend various clinics**, as proactively seeking them out will greatly aid your learning
- Ask how you can **help** with the running of the clinic, if this is appropriate
- **Never delay any aspect of the clinic** – if you have questions, arrange to ask them at a later time

# 16 Learning practical procedures

**Figure 16.1** Never events

**Surgical**

1. Wrong patient or wrong site of surgery
2. Wrong implant/prosthesis
3. Retained foreign object post-procedure

**Medication**

4. Mis-selection of a strong potassium containing solution
5. Wrong route administration of medication
6. Overdose of insulin due to abbreviations or incorrect device
7. Overdose of methotrexate for non-cancer treatment
8. Mis-selection of high strength midazolam during conscious sedation

**Mental health**

9. Failure to install functional collapsible shower or curtain rails

**General**

10. Falls from poorly restricted windows

Source: http://www.england.nhs.uk/wp-content/uploads/2015/03/never-evnts-list-15-16.pdf

**Figure 16.2** Types of simulations used at various medical schools

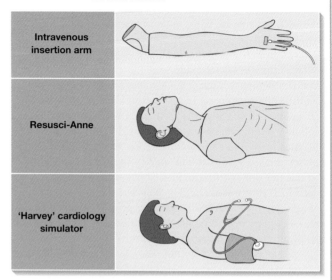

Intravenous insertion arm

Resusci-Anne

'Harvey' cardiology simulator

**Hints and Tips:**
- Always practise within your **competency**
- Ask for **feedback** to help with your learning on a patient – successful or otherwise
- **Remember** to **wash your hands** with the **six steps of hand hygiene,** at the **five moments of a clinical encounter**

**Figure 16.3** Stages of learning a procedure

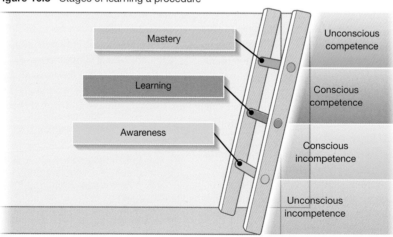

Mastery — Unconscious competence

Learning — Conscious competence

Awareness — Conscious incompetence

Unconscious incompetence

Source: Data from http://www.gordontraining.com, where employee Noel Burch developed 'learning stages model'.

# Practical procedures

A **practical procedure** is a key component of medicine – it enables **detection** (such as venepuncture to reveal a low potassium), **monitoring** (such as an arterial line to determine blood pressure) and **interventions** (such as an intravenous cannula to deliver fluids).

Historically, practical procedures were regarded with the mantra of 'see one, do one, teach one'. This had negative consequences for the patient and the student, and is now no longer regarded as an appropriate approach. Do not perform procedures that you do not feel **confident** or **competent** to perform. It is always better to ask for help when learning a new skill and to ensure that you are supervised adequately until you feel able to perform it **safely** and **effectively** on your own.

Trust your own instincts on when you feel capable of performing a procedure – do not feel pressured beyond your capabilities. You will be respected, not reprimanded, for **knowing your own limitations**. As with all areas of medicine, ensure the patient has been fully **identified** and has **given consent** before any procedures are undertaken.

**Never events** are events that **must not occur**, and incorrectly performing certain practical procedures, such as the incorrect route of administration of a medication, is included in the list of these events (Figure 16.1).

# Learning practical procedures

Much time is spent at medical school teaching the safe acquisition of skills for procedures. Most medical schools have **high-fidelity laboratories** for high-quality simulation to teach the skills safely (Figure 16.2). These skills are tested in practical examinations, either as part of the **objective structured clinical examinations** (OSCEs; see Chapter 32) or in a separate examination.

The list of procedures that a junior doctor must be competent in is clearly defined. You will be expected to be able to perform these on your first day on the job, so ensure you use your time at medical school to learn them. These are listed in the Foundation Programme websites, and on the GMC website.

**Cultivate good habits** early on. Ensure that you thoroughly wash your hands, according to the **six steps of hand hygiene**, at the **five moments of a clinical encounter** (see Chapter 7). Ensure that hands are **washed before** and **after** using gloves, as the gloves can act as a 'greenhouse' for bacterial growth.

There are many **opportunities** to practise these procedures. For example, you can offer to take blood samples during or after ward rounds. Spending time with an anaesthetist can provide valuable learning experiences in many areas, including cannulation. Going to specific departments of the hospital can be of benefit in learning particular procedures, such as spending time in Accident and Emergency for procedures such as ECGs.

# Stages of learning

There are various stages in learning a new procedure (Figure 16.3):
- Unconscious incompetence
- Conscious incompetence
- Conscious competence
- Unconscious competence.

In **unconscious incompetence**, you are unaware that you do not know what you are doing. In **conscious incompetence**, you

are aware that you are not able to perform the skill yet – and this is where learning begins. In **conscious competence**, you are aware that you are able to perform the procedure, and in **unconscious competence** you are able to naturally undertake the skill without being self-conscious.

# Performing a practical procedure

It takes **practice** to move through these stages of learning.

It is common to feel guilt about causing pain to patients when you are first learning some common procedures, such as venipuncture or cannulation. This can be minimised by ensuring that you have practised extensively in a **skills lab** prior to approaching a patient. When you do feel ready, ensure that you have the appropriate level of **supervision** as you:
- **Introduce** yourself
- Correctly **identify** the patient
- **Explain** the procedure to the patient
- Gain their **consent**
- Collect the appropriate **equipment**
- **Wash hands**
- Adhere to **local protocols**
- **Act confidently** as you perform the procedure, even if you are nervous.

# After the practical procedure

**Clean up immediately** after the procedure, including immediate disposal of **sharps** in **sharps bins**. These are often small and portable, and so should be collected for use prior to the procedure being performed. Remember that you are **responsible** for the disposal of the sharps that you use. Ensure that you never try to remove items from a sharps bin, and never insert your hands.

**Wash your hands** again after glove removal, and at the completion of the patient interaction. Ensure that clinical waste goes in the appropriate **clinical waste bin**.

Always ask for **feedback** from whoever has supervised you – be it a tutor, doctor, sister, nurse or fellow student – or from the patient. It may not be appropriate to do this immediately but most people will give feedback when they are able to.

Ensure that you **document** in the notes any attempts at a procedure, whether it failed or was successful. If you are unable to perform a procedure, ensure that you let someone know that you have been unsuccessful. The patient may be happy for you to try again later, or prefer that someone else attempt the procedure instead. Do not be embarrassed to ask their wishes, and then ensure that you respect them!

If you are unable to perform a procedure successfully, and you need someone else to do it for you, gestures such as collecting the required equipment for them can be helpful.

When **documenting** in the patient's notes, ensure that you include your **name**, your **designation** and to whom you **handed over** to if you were unsuccessful. Include other facts such as the date, time, consent, problems and how the patient was after the procedure. Include the sticker from equipment if there are any (such as from catheters). Ensure that you are familiar with **local protocols** and you record the procedure in the **appropriate area** (e.g. some Healthcare Trusts have a dedicated section for cannulae).

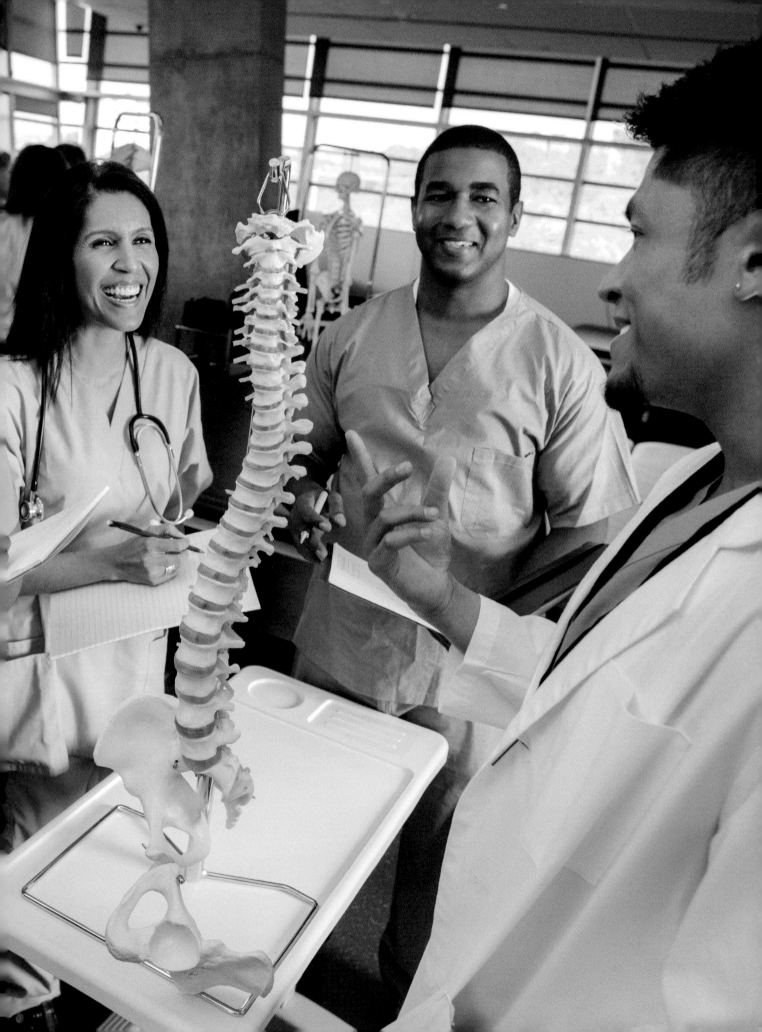

# Assessing a patient

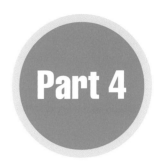

**Part 4**

## Chapters

# 17 Approaching a patient

**Figure 17.1  Approaching a patient**

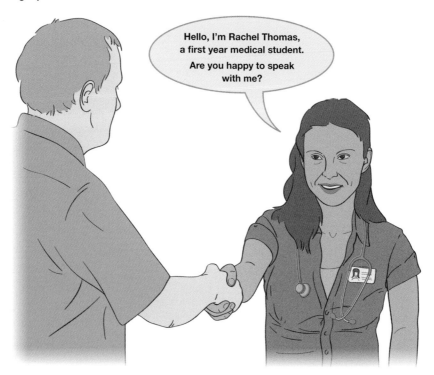

> **Did you know?**
>
> If you find it difficult to make and maintain eye contact with a patient, it can help to:
>
> • Relax, by taking a few deep breaths
> • Focus on just one eye, and then move to the other eye, after about 10 seconds
> • Focus on the space between their eyebrows, at the top of their nose
> • Look away from time to time, gently nodding while doing so
> • Practise maintain eye contact with your friends and family, or even with people on the television if you find it particularly difficult, so that you will feel more comfortable with patients, with whom you are less familiar

When you first start to see patients, the prospect may seem quite **daunting**. You may be excited, or you may feel ignorant and like a bit of an imposter.

However, it is important to remember to see any clinical interaction from the **patient's perspective**. They may be feeling anxious too. It may be their first time in hospital, or they may be extremely worried about why they are there. Some patients may be used to being in hospital. Some may already be **experts** in their own condition – so **listen** and **learn**, as they may be able to teach you more than you realise.

Do not be nervous about asking for **feedback** from patients. They may have interacted with many health professionals during their admission or over the course of their condition. As with all feedback, ensure that you **consider** it, and **act** on it where appropriate.

## Appearance

Remember that your patient may see you, and have formed an impression of you, **before** you have actually approached them. They may have seen you from the other end of the ward, for instance, before you are even aware of who or where they are. There is only one chance to make a **first impression**, so ensure that you make yours in a way that instils maximum **confidence** in you and in your skills – even if you are feeling less than maximally confident initially!

Your **body language** is important, as **non-verbal communication** is just as important as **verbal communication** – sometimes even more so (see Chapter 9).

Maintain **good eye contact** with your patient. This may feel unnatural at first, particularly if you are nervous. However, maintaining good eye contact assists in building **rapport** and **trust**. Eye contact should be 'natural', hence it also involves looking away from time to time. Intense staring can be intimidating, and can undermine rapport and connection just as much as insufficient eye contact.

Ensure that medical devices and other equipment are not between you and your patient, as this physical barrier can decrease rapport.

Stand straight, walk confidently and ensure that your posture is comfortable yet **attentive**. Avoid crossing your arms or putting your hands on your hips, as patients can interpret these gestures as indicating indifference or boredom.

Actions such as **handwashing** are important in the impression that you make on a patient. Perform this **in view** of the patient, so that they are reassured that you are setting an appropriate tone for the interaction. Ensure that you always use the **six steps** of hand hygiene, at the **five moments** of a clinical encounter (see Chapter 7). Make this a habit, from your first clinical interaction with a patient. It can be helpful to carry a small bottle of antiseptic gel with you. Many hospitals provide gel, or it can be bought for minimal cost at a pharmacy. Remember, however, that antiseptic gel does not kill all infectious organisms – for instance, *Clostridium difficile*, which is responsible for a particularly toxic form of gastroenteritis, requires washing with soap and water. Regular handwashing is one of the key aspects of **infection control**, as it breaks the **transmission cycle** of infection. Making it a **habit** now will also pay dividends during **exams** – where nerves can mean it is forgotten, and the result will be failing that area of the examination!

Ensure that you also extend these hygienic principles to your **stethoscope** – wipe it regularly with antiseptic wipes, as it is potentially another way of passing on infections.

Always dress appropriately for patient interactions, by wearing **smart**, **modest clothing**. It is common courtesy not to wear clothing that is too short, tight, low-cut, casual or dirty.

Hair should be tied back neatly if it is long, and nails should be kept short and clean (hair and nails are both infection risks). Local hospital policies vary on whether nail varnish is permitted. If varnish is worn, it is advisable to keep the tones neutral.

Remember you are reflecting your future profession, and hence should dress in a way **appropriate to this**. If you are unsure as to what is suitable, speak with your tutors or other healthcare professionals, or check the local guidelines and policies within your hospital.

Many hospitals have a **'bare below the elbows'** policy. Therefore, any long-sleeved shirts, sweaters or cardigans must be rolled up, and jewellery and watches removed. (There is often permission for a plain wedding band to be left on, depending upon local guidelines.) This is to facilitate adequate hand hygiene (see Chapter 7).

## Introducing yourself

'I'm just a medical student' is a commonly heard phrase in teaching hospitals. There is no need to apologise for being a student, as all doctors were one once. However, it is important to make this clear when first interacting with a patient.

Remember to **always introduce yourself**, and ensure that you have an official medical school name badge clearly visible to verify your identity (Figure 17.1): 'Hello, I am Rachel Thomas, a first year medical student. Are you happy to speak with me?'

Ensure that you then **fully identify** the patient, according to protocols.

## Consent

Always **gain consent** before talking to a patient (see Chapter 26). If they would prefer not to talk to you, thank them and leave them alone. They may wish to speak to you later – or not at all! Remember to respect their wishes.

---

**Hints and Tips:**
- Remember to ask for **feedback** from patients
- Always **introduce yourself**, and **ask for consent**, at the beginning of a clinical interaction
- Ensure that you **dress** and **act** in a way that is appropriate for your chosen profession

# 18 Approaching an unwell patient

**Figure 18.1** Vital signs recorded on an observation chart

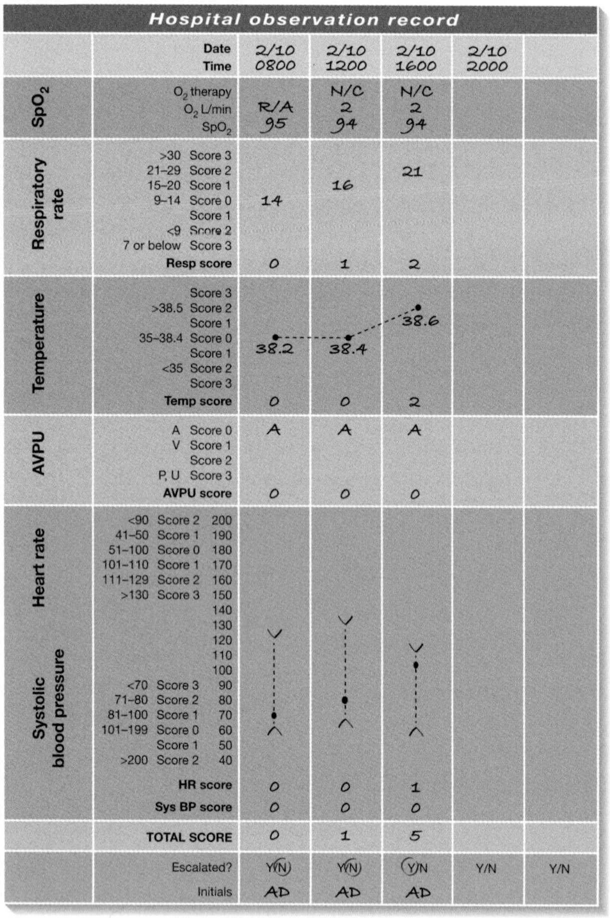

### Hospital observation record

|  |  | 2/10 0800 | 2/10 1200 | 2/10 1600 | 2/10 2000 |
|---|---|---|---|---|---|
| **Date** |  | | | | |
| **Time** |  | | | | |
| **SpO₂** | O₂ therapy | R/A | N/C | N/C | |
|  | O₂ L/min | | 2 | 2 | |
|  | SpO₂ | 95 | 94 | 94 | |
| **Respiratory rate** | >30 Score 3 | | | | |
|  | 21–29 Score 2 | | | 21 | |
|  | 15–20 Score 1 | | 16 | | |
|  | 9–14 Score 0 | 14 | | | |
|  | Score 1 | | | | |
|  | <9 Score 2 | | | | |
|  | 7 or below Score 3 | | | | |
|  | **Resp score** | 0 | 1 | 2 | |
| **Temperature** | Score 3 | | | | |
|  | >38.5 Score 2 | | | 38.6 | |
|  | Score 1 | | | | |
|  | 35–38.4 Score 0 | 38.2 | 38.4 | | |
|  | Score 1 | | | | |
|  | <35 Score 2 | | | | |
|  | Score 3 | | | | |
|  | **Temp score** | 0 | 0 | 2 | |
| **AVPU** | A Score 0 | A | A | A | |
|  | V Score 1 | | | | |
|  | Score 2 | | | | |
|  | P, U Score 3 | | | | |
|  | **AVPU score** | 0 | 0 | 0 | |
| **Heart rate** | <90 Score 2 200 | | | | |
|  | 41–50 Score 1 190 | | | | |
|  | 51–100 Score 0 180 | | | | |
|  | 101–110 Score 1 170 | | | | |
|  | 111–129 Score 2 160 | | | | |
|  | >130 Score 3 150 | | | | |
|  | 140 | | | | |
|  | 130 | | | | |
|  | 120 | | | | |
|  | 110 | | | | |
|  | 100 | | | | |
| **Systolic blood pressure** | 90 | | | | |
|  | <70 Score 3 80 | | | | |
|  | 71–80 Score 2 80 | | | | |
|  | 81–100 Score 1 70 | | | | |
|  | 101–199 Score 0 60 | | | | |
|  | Score 1 50 | | | | |
|  | >200 Score 2 40 | | | | |
|  | **HR score** | 0 | 0 | 1 | |
|  | **Sys BP score** | 0 | 0 | 0 | |
| **TOTAL SCORE** |  | 0 | 1 | 5 | |
| Escalated? |  | Y/N | Y/N | Y/N | Y/N | Y/N |
| Initials |  | AD | AD | AD | | |

Source: *Thomas R. Practical Medical Procedures at a Glance (2015).*
*Reproduced with permission of John Wiley & Sons Ltd.*

**Figure 18.2** Modified early warning system (MEWS)

| Score | 3 | 2 | 1 | 0 | 1 | 2 | 3 |
|---|---|---|---|---|---|---|---|
| **Systolic BP** | <70 | 70–80 | 81–100 | 101–100 | | ≥200 | |
| **Heart rate (bpm)** | | 40 | 41–100 | 51–100 | 101–110 | 111–29 | ≥130 |
| **Respiratory rate (bpm)** | | <9 | | 9–14 | 15–20 | 21–9 | >30 |
| **Temperature (°C)** | | <35 | | 35.0–38.4 | | ≥38.5 | |
| **AVPU score** | | | | Alert | Reactive to voice | Reacting to pain | Unresponsive |

Source: *Subbe et al. Q J Med, 2001; 94: 521–526.*
*Reproduced with permission of Oxford University Press.*

**Figure 18.3** The Glasgow Coma Scale

| Behaviour | Response | Score |
|---|---|---|
| **Eye opening response** | Spontaneous | 4 |
|  | To Speech | 3 |
|  | To pain | 2 |
|  | No response | 1 |
| **Best verbal response** | Oriented to time, place, and person | 5 |
|  | Confused | 4 |
|  | Inappropriate words | 3 |
|  | Incomprehensible sounds | 2 |
|  | No response | 1 |
| **Best motor response** | Obeys commands | 6 |
|  | Moves to localised pain | 5 |
|  | Flexion withdrawal from pain | 4 |
|  | Abnormal flexion (decorticate) | 3 |
|  | Abnormal extension (decerebrate) | 2 |
|  | No response | 1 |
| **Total score:** | *Best response* | 15 |
|  | *Totally unresponsive* | 3 |

Source: *Data from http://www.glasgowcomascale.org*

**Figure 18.4** The AVPU scale

| **A** | Alert |
|---|---|
| **V** | Verbal stimuli |
| **P** | Painful stimuli |
| **U** | Unresponsive |

**Figure 18.5** ABC on a patient

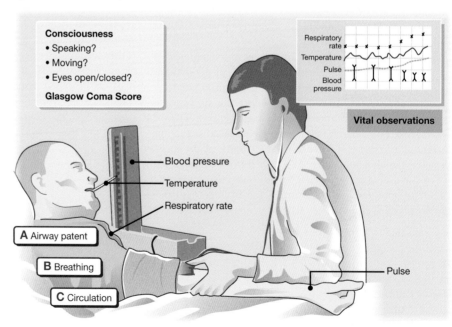

**Consciousness**
- Speaking?
- Moving?
- Eyes open/closed?

**Glasgow Coma Score**

Respiratory rate
Temperature
Pulse
Blood pressure

**Vital observations**

Blood pressure
Temperature
Respiratory rate

Pulse

**A** Airway patent
**B** Breathing
**C** Circulation

## Approaching an unwell patient on the ward

When you will commence seeing patients during your course varies depending on the curriculum of your medical school. Remember that you should always have a **low threshold** for **seeking help** if you are worried about a patient. A patient's condition can **deteriorate quickly**, so ensure that you are aware of the relevant **national and local guidelines and protocols** and always be **alert** to signs indicating deterioration. **Recognising** the point at which you should seek help is an important skill to learn.

This chapter is written as a **basic guide** on how to help you to start 'thinking like a doctor' when managing an unwell patient. As a medical student (and even as a doctor at times) you are yet to acquire the knowledge or skills needed to manage an unwell patient. Thus, you **should call for help immediately**, and highlight the fact that you are a medical student and that calling the doctor is the best course of action. **Get the patient the most appropriate help as early as possible.** Consider shadowing the team that subsequently becomes involved with this patient if this is appropriate. You will then be better prepared for similar situations in the future.

When you approach the patient's bedside, introduce yourself, identify them correctly, ask them how they are feeling, and if they consent to seeing you. With this brief general exchange, you can establish if the patient is **alert, orientated** and also their **general appearance**. This will give you an idea of what type of interaction you can have with the patient and whether they need **urgent senior help** such as a doctor or even a **crash call**.

While at the bedside, look at the **observation chart** and the **trend** of these observations (Figure 18.1). There are various **early warning systems**, such as the modified early warning system (MEWS), that can help to identify patients as they become unwell, because they trigger by **trends** or **critical values** on their observation charts (Figure 18.2).

If a patient is unwell or deteriorating, seek a **doctor**, **crash call** and/or start **basic life support/advanced life support according to guidelines** as appropriate. While the doctors are treating the patient, start learning how to manage an acutely unwell patient by observing and helping as appropriate. Depending on the situation, the doctor may:

- Clarify why they were called, and what the **clinical situation** is
- Look at the patient's **clinical notes**, to help establish a **background** and **timeline**
- Look at the most **recent plan** for the patient
- Look at the patient's investigation **results** such as blood tests or images such as X-rays or scans
- Look at **vital observations**, and establish **trends**
- Look at the **drug chart**, and determine what drugs the patient is on and what they have been on
- **Management** so far, including any recent procedures/operations, any recent medications/fluids that have been started or changed.

## Assessing an unwell patient on the ward

A doctor may use various methods to assess a patient, some of which are covered here. The treating clinician may:

- Try to obtain a **brief, focused history** from the patient (if possible), and from staff or family caring for the patient, including asking if anything has changed recently or acutely.
- **Look** at the patient from the end of the bed for a **global view** of them and to identify **respiratory rate**, **work of breathing** and the **Glasgow Coma Score** (GCS) as an indication of consciousness (Figure 18.3). Alternatively, AVPU can be used (Figure 18.4).
- Perform a **focused examination**, assessing the **ABC** steps thoroughly, as well as any **other systems** that have been involved (e.g. in a post-laparotomy patient it is important to examine the abdomen)

(Figure 18.5). This should be performed according to the current appropriate **local** and **national guidelines** such as those of the Resuscitation Council UK (https://www.resus.org.uk), so ensure that you are always familiar with these.

The following basic points are included to help start guiding your initial stages of learning, and are not exhaustive.

**A is for Airway** Is there any compromise? Can they talk? Is there a cough, stridor, wheeze or tracheostomy?

**B is for Breathing** Examine the chest. Are they breathing, and if so, how fast? Take the respiratory rate (RR) and sats. Is there increased work of breathing or is it in an unusual pattern? Are there any focal signs? (Consider giving oxygen if appropriate.)

**C is for Circulation** Examine the heart. Take the heart rate (HR), noting volume/irregularity, and blood pressure (BP), noting postural drops. Check the peripheral circulation with the capillary refill time (CRT). Are they warm or cool? Do they look cyanosed? Consider looking at the jugular venous pressure (JVP), the legs for oedema, and the calves for tenderness. (Consider gaining IV access and giving IV fluids if appropriate; see Chapter 31).

**D is for Disability** Take the temperature and the patient's blood sugar level, assess the GCS or AVPU, check for confusion, check pupillary responses. Is the patient in pain? Consider focused neurological examination if indicated.

**E is for Exposure** Consider exposure and examination of the skin.

As a learning guide and useful mnemonic or aide-memoire, F–I can be used to remind you of further possible considerations, which are include, but are not limited to:

**F is for Fluids** What is the patient's intake and output? Are they passing urine? Have they been given IV fluids – if so how much and what type? Look at the most recent U+Es and the trend. Is there a catheter – and if so, is it blocked?

**G is for Gastrointestinal** Consider examination of the abdomen including a *per rectum* (PR) examination if indicated. Have their bowels opened recently? Any drains in situ?

**H is for Haematology** Look at the most recent blood results. Is there any evidence of blood loss?

**I is for Infection** Are they on any antibiotics? Check their inflammatory markers, recent culture results and send for further blood tests if indicated.

## Considering an unwell patient

Formulate your own **differential diagnosis** as you are observing the doctors, based on what information you have so far. What do you think is going on? If you do not know do not panic, go back to your ABC and think it through.

Remember to consider **your own** needs as well. Seeing an unwell patient or a patient whom you know is deteriorating in condition, or dying, is **emotionally challenging**. If you feel you need to talk to someone about it, speak to your supervisor or try to have a **de-brief** session with the doctors who were involved. This can both provide you with **support**, as well as **aid learning** for future similar situations.

You may also be able to **help** in practical ways, assisting the doctors as they manage the unwell patient. This can include getting gloves or equipment, taking arterial blood gas (ABG) results to the analyser or helping to gain venous access and taking blood samples. Listen to what your seniors are asking of you, and do that which is within your capabilities.

**Hints and Tips:**
**Ask for help immediately if you are concerned about a patient**

# 19 Taking a history

**Figure 19.1** Some aspects to consider in a systems enquiry

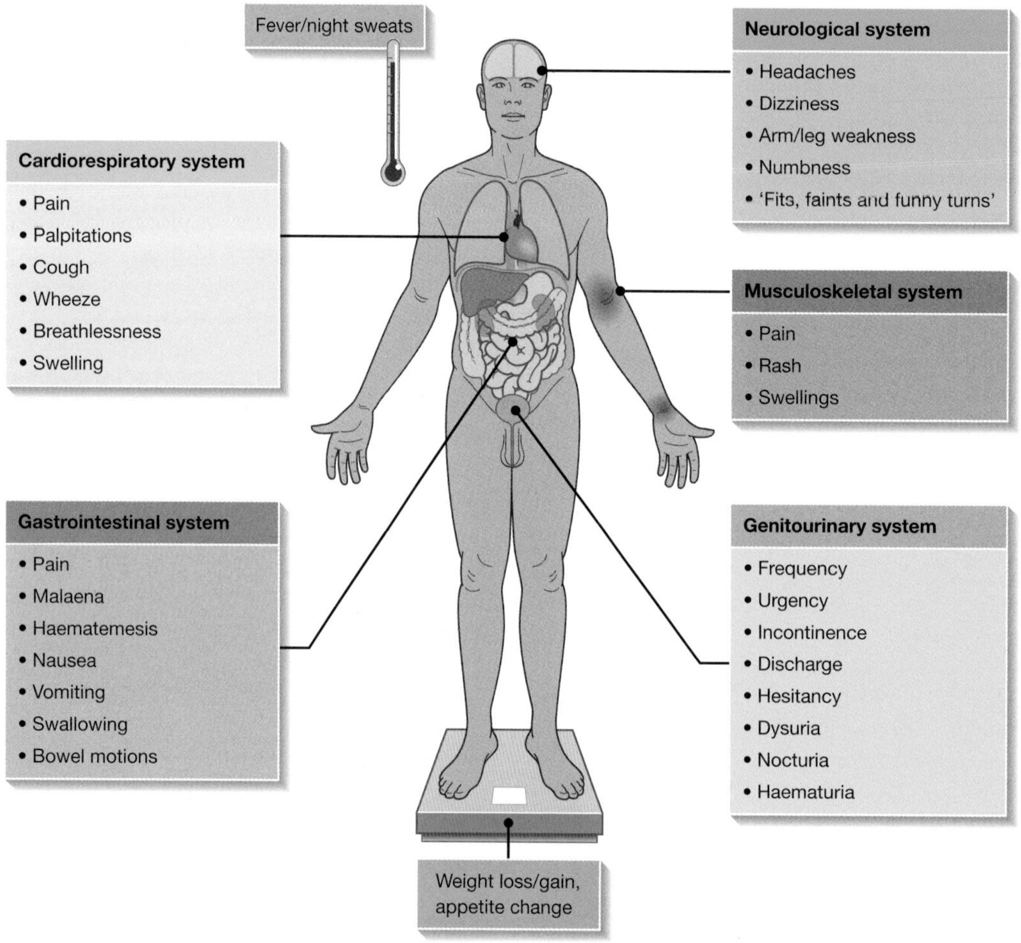

Fever/night sweats

**Neurological system**
- Headaches
- Dizziness
- Arm/leg weakness
- Numbness
- 'Fits, faints and funny turns'

**Cardiorespiratory system**
- Pain
- Palpitations
- Cough
- Wheeze
- Breathlessness
- Swelling

**Musculoskeletal system**
- Pain
- Rash
- Swellings

**Gastrointestinal system**
- Pain
- Malaena
- Haematemesis
- Nausea
- Vomiting
- Swallowing
- Bowel motions

**Genitourinary system**
- Frequency
- Urgency
- Incontinence
- Discharge
- Hesitancy
- Dysuria
- Nocturia
- Haematuria

Weight loss/gain, appetite change

**Hints and Tips:**

Ask the patient about their **'ICE'**:
- Their **ideas** about what is causing their illness
- Their **concerns** about what may happen
- Their **expectations** of their treatment

Listen carefully to the patient, as they will often provide valuable and **correct insight** into their condition.

**Did you know?**

In the **social history**, you should record
- **Alcohol** consumed in **units per week**: (unit = 10ml of pure alcohol, and varies with strength and quantity, e.g. 250ml of 4% beer or 25ml of 40% whiskey)
- **Cigarettes** smoked in **pack years**: (pack years = number of years they have smoked × number of cigarettes per day/number of cigarettes in a pack)

## What is a history?

A history is also referred to as a **patient history**, **medical history** or a **patient case history**. It is often abbreviated to **Hx** in patient notes. It involves asking **specific questions** in order to gain the maximum amount of **information**, so that you can make an **accurate diagnosis**. You will spend a lot of time at medical school learning to take histories, as they are a key aspect of a doctor's job. Devote time to learning the appropriate sections that you need to cover, as histories are easier to take when you can actually listen to the patient, rather than when you are trying to remember what you need to ask next!

Do write down as much as you need to, while you are speaking with the patient. It may be appropriate to acknowledge this to the patient with, 'Are you happy for me to write down some points as we speak?' You will need to learn to **document fully** your completed history and examination, so writing it up as you go or afterwards will depend on your personal preference.

It can be frustrating when first learning how to take histories, as the information may not be in the standard order – it may seem like it is in the 'wrong' order! But rest assured that with practice you will be able to re-order and present it more easily, and remember that you are not the first student to feel like this!

*Medical School at a Glance*, First Edition. Rachel K. Thomas © 2017 John Wiley & Sons, Ltd. Published 2017 by John Wiley & Sons, Ltd.

**Practice makes perfect.** Try taking histories from **many sources** – family, friends, peers and patients. Becoming comfortable asking people about their past and current circumstances can be challenging, but practice will help.

## Taking a history

As with any patient interaction, always **introduce yourself, identify** the patient and ask if the patient **agrees** to talk with you in order to gain **consent** (see Chapter 26). Ensure that there is as much **privacy** as possible, and that the patient is **comfortable.**

While there are specific areas that you will need to cover, try to ask 'open questions' whenever you can. These are questions without a 'yes' or 'no' answer. It is acceptable to ask more 'closed questions' in order to clarify any points of confusion of facts, but try to use open questions as frequently as possible, particularly when you are first speaking with the patient.

Try not to ask 'leading questions', where you imply the answer. For instance, 'Is your pain sharp or stabbing?' when in fact it may be dull.

Remember that you can use **different sources** of information to expand your history, such as additional facts from **family members** or **carers**. Ensure that you maintain the patient's confidentiality in these cases, and that you do not disclose anything (accidentally or otherwise) without the patient's expressed consent.

Always ask the patient if they have any **ideas** on what is the matter with them. You will be surprised to find how often they are right!

## Components of a history

A history is divided up into **several sections:**
- Presenting complaint
- History of presenting complaint
- Past medical history
- Drug history
- Family history
- Social history
- Systems enquiry.

The **presenting complaint** (PC) is the main reason that the patient has sought medical attention, and should be recorded in the **patient's own words.** For instance, they have come to hospital for 'stomach ache' rather than 'central abdominal pains'.

The **history of presenting complaint** (HxPC or HPC) is the background behind the presenting complaint. Ensure that you use open questions here, such as 'Can you please tell me more about your . . .'.

**Mnemonics** can help with remembering specific questions. For instance, to characterise pain, the following questions (which can be remembered as SOCRATES) could be asked:
- Site (e.g. arm, leg, head, abdomen, back)
- Onset (e.g. sudden, days, week, months, years)
- Characteristic (e.g. dull, stabbing, sharp, wringing)
- Radiation (e.g. to the jaw, down the limb)
- Additional symptoms (e.g. fever, nausea)
- Timing (e.g. at night, after movement)
- Exacerbating factors (e.g. movement, temperature)
- Severity out of 10 (where 10 is the worst pain imaginable)

When using mnemonics, do not write them in the patient notes – ensure you write the full words that the letter represents.

Try to rule in or rule out the **life-threatening causes** of the PC, and ask about **risk factors**. For instance, with a sudden onset chest pain, you should ask about aspects such as recent periods of immobility or air travel in an effort to exclude a pulmonary embolus (PE).

The **past medical history** (PMHx or PMH) also includes past surgical history. It can be helpful to ask about specific conditions (commonly remembered by the mnemonic MJTHREADS):
- Myocardial infarction
- Jaundice
- Tuberculosis
- Hypertension
- Rheumatoid arthritis
- Epilepsy
- Asthma
- Diabetes mellitus
- Stroke.

Remember to ask about any hospital admissions, and what happened during them such as any ITU admissions.

The **drug history** (DHx or DH) includes all medications that the patient is taking, including contraceptive medications, alternative or complementary medications, and medications that do not require prescription (known as over-the-counter or OTC medications). Ask also about any **allergies** to medications or foods. If they have none, document **no known drug allergies** (NKDA).

The **family history** (FHx or FH) involves asking about any conditions that run in the family, such as cancer.

At first, you may feel uncomfortable asking about the **social history** (SHx or SH), as it involves questions that are beyond a normal social context. However, it is a key part of the history, as it focuses on how the patient is **managing at home**. Remember to be 'matter of fact' in asking these questions. It can be helpful if you explain that you are 'asking these questions to gauge how you are getting along at home'. Ask about who they live with, their type of home, if they need any help at home to do **activities of daily living** (ADLs).

Ensure you ask about **smoking, alcohol** consumption and **illicit drug consumption**.

A **systems review** (Sys Rv, Syx, Sys Rx) or **functional enquiry** is a helpful **catch-all** at the end of the history to help you ask anything that you may have forgotten earlier on, and to help you clarify the diagnosis by asking about other body systems (Figure 19.1).

## Completing the history

After you have asked all the components of the history, ensure that you give the patient time to ask any **questions**. Ask the patient if there is anything that they feel you have not covered or that they are worried about, as you may have **missed** one of their key symptoms or concerns.

If a patient has questions you cannot answer, ask a senior to discuss them with the patient. Try to present any patient that you have taken a history from. You can **present** them to fellow students or doctors, and remember to specifically ask for **feedback** on how to improve this important skill.

# 20 Examining a patient

**Figure 20.1** Basic examination principles

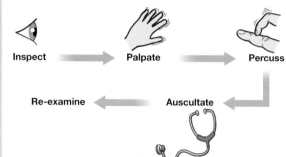

Inspect → Palpate → Percuss

Re-examine ← Auscultate ←

**Hints and Tips:**

- Remember to ask for **consent**, and to maintain the patient's **dignity**
- If a patient asks you to **stop**, do so without hesitation!
- Ensure adequate **hand hygiene**, using the 6 steps at the 5 moments of a clinical encounter
- Try to **present your findings** to a friend or colleague

Source: *Davey P. (ed) Medicine at a Glance, 4th edn (2014)*
*Reproduced with permission of John Wiley & Sons Ltd.*

**Figure 20.2** Aspects to consider in examining the patient's systems

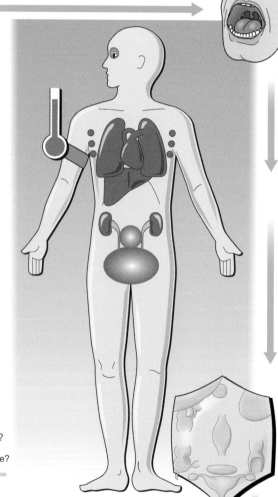

**Blood pressure**
- Supine
- Standing

**Radial pulse**
- Rate
- Rhythm
- Volume
- Character

**Hands**
- Clubbing
- Splinters
- Palmar erythema

**Vital observations**
- Pulse
- BP
- Temperature
- Respiratory rate

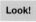Look!

**Is the patient unwell?**
- Is there anaemia, cyanosis, jaundice?
- Is the patient well hydrated, nourished?
- Any obvious signs of endocrine disease?

**Mouth and tongue**
- Cyanosis
- Dry mucous membranes
- Pigmentation

**Neck**
- Carotid pulse
- JVP
- Goitre
- Lymph nodes

**Chest**
- Scars
- Chest movements
- Respiratory rate
- Tracheal position
- Chest expansion
- Apex beat
- Heaves/thrills
- Auscultate heart
- Percuss/auscultate front of chest
- Examine breasts/axillae
- Sit forwards:
  - sacral oedema
  - spine
  - percuss/auscultate back of chest

**Abdomen**
- Inspect
- Palpate
- Percuss
- Auscultate
- Examine for:
  Liver, spleen, kidneys, aorta, herniae, lymph nodes

**Legs**
- Oedema
- Rashes
- Peripheral pulses

**Neurology**
- Conscious level
- Speech
- Memory
- Orientation
- Gait
- Limbs
- Eyes
- Cranial nerves

Source: *Gleadle J. History and Clinical Examination at a Glance, 3rd edn (2012).*
*Reproduced with permission of John Wiley & Sons Ltd.*

You will perform **physical examinations** on many patients while in medical school, and countless others during your career as a practising clinician. It can help your learning to pair with another student, **alternating** who examines the patient and who observes and provides feedback and to practise on each other.

There is a **'performance'** element to a patient examination, in trying to appear calm while trying to remember where to move to next in your examination. This may be particularly evident in your medical school assessments. However, you will become more **proficient** as you perform more examinations. You will soon stop focusing on what to do next, and start **recognising signs** and piecing them together while examining the patient.

The aim of this chapter is to help you provide a framework for some common principles in the examinations. It is important to use a **methodical framework** for each body system. Components are examined in a **specific order**, and you should not deviate from this order, or you can miss something important.

There are different ways to examine a patient in different situations – for example, in an **emergency** start with **ABC**. A **general clerking exam** when you first see a patient in hospital will involve looking at all the systems together. Usually, when learning, you will be expected to cover each body system in its entirety, but only one system at a time.

Before starting to examine a patient, put yourself in their shoes. How would you feel if someone you have only just met wants to feel your hands or touch your stomach, particularly if you are in pain? What would you prefer if you were going to be examined? Think about the patient's **privacy, dignity** and **comfort**. Remember, it is a **privilege** for you, as a medical student, to examine someone, as you are doing it for your own **learning only.**

## Before touching the patient

**Introduce** yourself to the patient after fully identifying them (see Chapter 17).

**Explain** what you are going to do, for example, 'Mr Jones I would like to examine you now, this would involve examining your hands, arms and face, and listening to your chest. This would mean that I would need you to be partly undressed for some of the examination. Would that be all right?' Gain **consent** before proceeding (see Chapter 26).

Consider having a **chaperone** present – because either the patient or you would prefer to have one. It is advisable to always have a chaperone present during intimate examinations.

Consider to what degree the patient should **undress** for the examination, and with what the patient would be comfortable. Have a sheet or a blanket to **maintain dignity** when performing the examination, covering an area after your have examined it.

Consider the lighting, space and equipment available. Common pieces of **equipment** required are a stethoscope, tendon hammer, ophthalmoscope, saturations probe, blood pressure cuff, measuring tape or torch, so try to collect the necessary equipment before starting the examination.

Types of hospital beds vary, even within the same ward. A quick and easy filter for medical school examiners to reveal which students have been on the wards frequently is by testing who can easily flatten the bed or lower its sides!

**Wash your hands** before you approach the patient (see Chapter 7).

Each examination starts with **inspection** (Figure 20.1). From the end of the bed observe:

• *The bedside* Are there any medications (e.g. inhalers, food supplements, pills, lotions) around the bed? Does the patient have a catheter or any drains and what is draining (e.g. blood, urine, faeces, serous fluid, empty bag)? Any sputum or urine pots by the bedside? Any machines the patient is connected to (e.g. dialysis)?

• *The patient* Are they comfortable? Is there anything you can do to make them more comfortable? Observe any equipment that the patient has, such as for monitoring (e.g. saturations probe, heart rate)? Are they on oxygen or fluids? Does the patient have any obvious peripheral or central lines, or feeding tubes (e.g. nasogastric tube)?

In an exam or assessment situation, it is advisable to **comment** on what is present or absent in these areas as you observe them, to avoid forgetting to comment on them after.

## Contacting the patient

Every examination differs, but all are based on **similar principles**. After **inspection**, generally you will move to **feeling**, known as **palpating**. After this, you will generally proceed to **gently tapping (percussing)** and **listening (auscultating)** to areas of the patient which are components of the body systems (Figure 20.2).

When palpating and percussing, ensure that you do not cause the patient any **discomfort** or harm.

Anatomically, many examinations **start peripherally** and **move centrally** – for example, you may start at the patient's finger nails. Then you can move to the patient's hands and systematically work your way up from their hands, noticing the appropriate components for the relevant systems (e.g. abdominal, respiratory or cardiovascular systems).

Other examinations follow a slightly **different format** (e.g. the cranial nerves). Many medical students find examination of the cranial nerves challenging because it is long-winded and requires a level of understanding of neuro-anatomy in order to decipher the signs!

Other general principles include comparing **'like for like'** (e.g. testing the power of the patient's thumb against the power of your own thumb), and **'symmetry'** (e.g. comparing each side of the chest in the same location while the patient inhales), which will help you to start noticing **abnormal signs.**

During the examination, ensure that you are not rushed, if possible. If you are having difficulty identifying any abnormalities, try determining the 'normalities', and then distinguish what is different. But do not take so long that the patient becomes uncomfortable. Also remember that most medical school assessments have a time limit (such as 7 minutes) during which time you must complete the examination.

## After examining the patient

After you have completed your examination, thank the patient, ask if there is anything that you can do for them and check that they are **comfortable**. Offer to help **them dress again**, and to return to the position they were originally in.

If appropriate, ask the patient if they have any **feedback** for you.

Ensure that you **wash** your hands, clean your stethoscope and dispose of any equipment in the appropriate clinical bins.

Practise **presenting** your findings to a colleague (or your student 'pair') and ask for feedback.

# 21 Assessing a patient's hydration

**Figure 21.1** Fluid distribution in an average adult

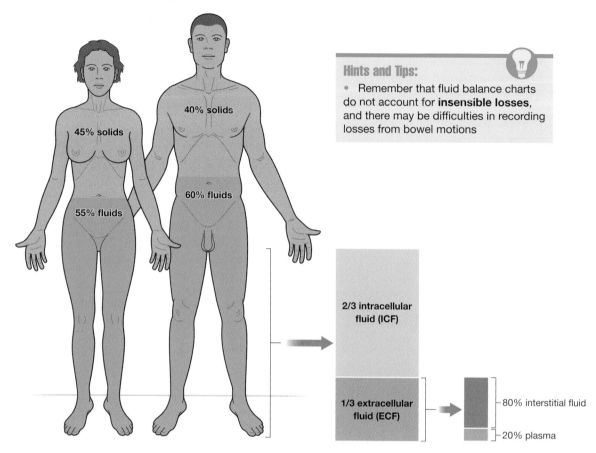

45% solids

55% fluids

40% solids

60% fluids

**Hints and Tips:**
• Remember that fluid balance charts do not account for **insensible losses**, and there may be difficulties in recording losses from bowel motions

2/3 intracellular fluid (ICF)

1/3 extracellular fluid (ECF)

80% interstitial fluid

20% plasma

**Figure 21.2** A fluid balance chart

Name: A. Patient    Date: 28/03/17    Fluid restriction: Yes ☐ ___ mls  No ☑    24 hr Target balances: +ve ___ mls  -ve ___ mls

| Time | Input | | | | | | Output | | | | | | | Initials |
|---|---|---|---|---|---|---|---|---|---|---|---|---|---|---|
| | Oral intake | External feed | IV fluids | Other | Other | Total input | Urine | Vomit | Bowels | Drain | Drain | Other | Total output | |
| 01:00 | | | | | | | | | | | | | | |
| 02:00 | | | | | | | | | | | | | | |
| 03:00 | | | | | | | | | | | | | | |
| 04:00 | | | | | | | | | | | | | | |
| 05:00 | | | | | | | | | | | | | | |
| 06:00 | | | | | | | | 200 | | | | | | RT |
| 07:00 | | | | | | | | | | | | | | |
| 08:00 | 250 | | | | | | | | | | | | | |
| 09:00 | | | 125 | | | | 20 | | | | | | | RT |
| 10:00 | | | 125 | | | | 10 | | Diarrhoea ? volume | | | | | RT |
| 11:00 | | | 125 | | | | 10 | | | | | | | RT |
| 12:00 | | | 125 | | | | 50 | | Diarrhoea ? volume | | | | | RT |
| 13:00 | | | 125 | | | | 10 | | | | | | | RT |
| 14:00 | | | 125 | | | | 15 | | | | | | | RT |
| 15:00 | | | 125 | | | | 25 | | | | | | | RT |
| 16:00 | | | 125 | | | | 40 | | | 50 | | | | T.C |
| 17:00 | | | 250 | | | | 10 | 100 | | | | | | T.C |
| 18:00 | | | 250 | | | | 25 | | | | | | | T.C |
| 19:00 | | | 250 | | | | 75 | | | | | | | T.C |
| 20:00 | | | 250 | | | | 50 | | | | | | | T.C |
| 21:00 | | | 125 | | | | 80 | 200 | | | | | | T.C |
| 22:00 | | | 125 | | | | 100 | | | | | | | T.C |
| 23:00 | | | 125 | | | | 110 | | | | | | | T.C |
| 00:00 | | | 125 | | | | 120 | | | | | | | T.C |
| Cumulative total | 250 | 0 | 2500 | | | 2750 | 750 | 500 | | 50 | | | 1300 | |

*Medical School at a Glance*, First Edition. Rachel K. Thomas © 2017 John Wiley & Sons, Ltd. Published 2017 by John Wiley & Sons, Ltd.

Assessing the hydration of a patient is **important** and should be part of a routine assessment. This part of the assessment can be particularly challenging.

**Renal team doctors** are **experts** at assessing hydration, and spending time with them while in medical school can be enormously beneficial for your learning.

For a patient to be **adequately hydrated** there has to be:

- Enough fluid (blood volume) to perfuse all the necessary organs (no signs of end-organ compromise).
- The fluid has to be in the right space (in the intravascular compartment rather than the extravascular compartment).

When considering **total body water**, it is important to think about:

- The **compartments** of total body water (Figure 21.1)
- Where total body water comes from (**intake** in the form of fluid, **re-uptake** of water particularly from the gastrointestinal tract and the kidneys and a minority from cell reactions)
- Where fluid is **lost**: urine, stool (usually very little unless there is profound diarrhoea), sweat and lungs.

Fluid losses can be divided into **sensible losses** (losses that we can easily measure, e.g. urine output) and **insensible losses** (e.g. water lost from the skin or the lungs).

## Patients at risk of dehydration

When considering a patient's hydration status, remember that some patients are at higher risk of **dehydration**:

- Patients whose **current medical problem** includes fluid loss (e.g. a diarrhoeal illness, haemorrhage where fluid loss is the primary problem, diabetes – insipidus or mellitus – and patients with a 'third spacing' of fluid, e.g. pancreatitis or infection/sepsis)
- Those who are **dependent** on others for eating and drinking
- Those who have **communication barriers** (including patients in intensive care who are sedated and paralysed)
- Children
- Patients with cardiac or neurological dysfunction, as a result of being on multiple diuretics or with injuries affecting their thirst sensation, respectively.

## Assessing a patient's hydration

There is **no single gold standard test** for determining a patient's hydration status. Take a **thorough history**, including:

- How many times a day they have passed **urine**
- **Colour** of the urine
- How many times they have opened their **bowels**
- **Consistency** of the stool
- Recent **travel**.

Then assess hydration using various components.

### 1 Charts

- *Observation charts* Look at the patient's observation chart. What is their heart rate and blood pressure? Tachycardia and hypotension can indicate depleted intravascular volume. Do they have an elevated temperature? A high temperature means there may be more insensible water loss from the skin. Sometimes the patient can have a lying and standing blood pressure drop (orthostatic hypotension) – a difference of more than 22 mmHg in systolic or 10 mmHg in diastolic blood pressure when changing their position – which can have various causes including dehydration.
- *Fluid balance charts* The fluid balance chart (Figure 21.2) documents the patient's **input** (i.e. fluid they take in) and **output** (usually measurements of urine and documentation of whether the bowels were opened and the consistency of the stool). This chart provides an estimate of overall fluid balance (fluid input – fluid output = overall fluid balance). A **negative balance** means that the patient is **losing** more fluid than they are taking in. A **positive balance** means that the patient is **retaining** fluid.
- *Daily weights* Some patients are weighed in the early mornings. This is useful as a **surrogate marker** of overall hydration.

### 2 Patient

- Ask the patient if they are thirsty.
- Feel the skin turgor, examine for capillary refill time, look at their mucous membranes (are they dry?) Does the patient have sunken eyes?
- Feel the pulse: volume (is it thready?) Is the patient tachycardic?
- Feel the temperature of their hands and arms. In severe dehydration or hypovolaemia, blood is shunted from the peripheral circulation to the central circulation, and thus they can feel cool.
- You can also examine the veins (e.g. examine the jugular venous pressure as a surrogate marker to see how 'filled' the patient is).

### 3 Tests

- *Urinalysis* Look at the **colour** of the urine (dark or light). Dark yellow urine suggests that the urine is more concentrated, indicating the patient might be intravascularly fluid depleted. **Urine specific gravity** can be used as a surrogate marker for hydration. **Urine osmolality** can also be used and the **paired measurements** of **urine and plasma osmolality** are often used to further assess fluid status.
- *Blood tests* **Renal function tests**, and their **trends**, include looking at electrolytes (sodium, potassium), renal function surrogate markers (creatinine and estimated glomerular filtration rate (eGFR), with urea often included). For example, an elevated urea suggests dehydration. Beware, however, as there are other causes for an elevated urea (e.g. digested blood in an upper gastrointestinal bleed). Creatinine and/or eGFR trends (rising creatinine, reduction in eGFR) indicate impending acute kidney injury, while rising sodium suggests dehydration.

**Plasma osmolality** (Posm) is a measurement of the extracellular fluid osmolality and can give an indication of hydration status. Posm is usually 285–295 mOsm/kg. An elevated Posm suggests dehydration. Posm can be estimated by $(2 \times Na) + (2 \times K) +$ glucose + urea.

- *Invasive tests* In intensive care, invasive measurements (e.g. invasive arterial blood pressure monitoring, central venous pressure monitoring) help to assess whether the patient is 'underfilled' or 'overfilled'.

## Managing dehydration

The management of dehydration depends on its cause and the patient's overall clinical status. In many cases, it involves giving the patient fluid either **orally** or **through a vein**, and should be carried out according to **local** and **national protocols**.

# 22 Assessing a patient's nutrition

**Figure 22.1** The dynamic integration of various factors involved in nutritional status

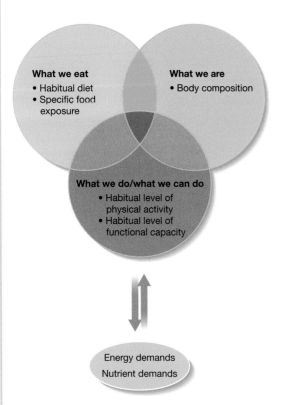

**What we eat**
- Habitual diet
- Specific food exposure

**What we are**
- Body composition

**What we do/what we can do**
- Habitual level of physical activity
- Habitual level of functional capacity

Energy demands
Nutrient demands

**Figure 22.2** Routes of nutritional support

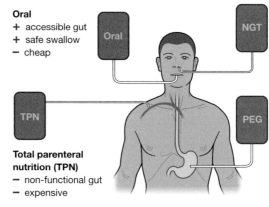

**Oral**
+ accessible gut
+ safe swallow
− cheap

**Nasogastric tube (NGT)**
+ accessible gut
− unsafe swallow
− inadequate oral intake

**Percutaneous enterogastroscopy (PEG)**
+ accessible gut functional GI system
− unsafe swallow
− long-term enteral requirements

**Total parenteral nutrition (TPN)**
− non-functional gut
− expensive

**Hints and Tips:**
- Spend time with **dietitians** to learn more about nutrition
- Remember to ask about **weight loss/gain** when learning to take a **history**
- Remember that **nutritional support** can improve the **patient's recovery rate**
- It is very important to **observe NBM signs**
- Remember that **malnutrition** affects both **mortality** and **morbidity**

**Figure 22.3** Refeeding syndrome

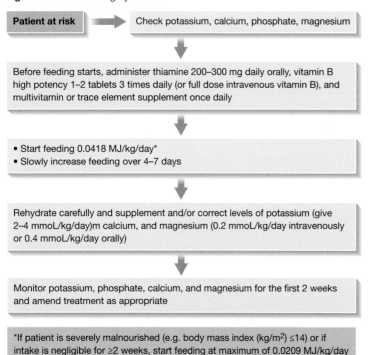

**Patient at risk** ➡ Check potassium, calcium, phosphate, magnesium

Before feeding starts, administer thiamine 200–300 mg daily orally, vitamin B high potency 1–2 tablets 3 times daily (or full dose intravenous vitamin B), and multivitamin or trace element supplement once daily

- Start feeding 0.0418 MJ/kg/day*
- Slowly increase feeding over 4–7 days

Rehydrate carefully and supplement and/or correct levels of potassium (give 2–4 mmoL/kg/day)m calcium, and magnesium (0.2 mmoL/kg/day intravenously or 0.4 mmoL/kg/day orally)

Monitor potassium, phosphate, calcium, and magnesium for the first 2 weeks and amend treatment as appropriate

*If patient is severely malnourished (e.g. body mass index (kg/m²) ≤14) or if intake is negligible for ≥2 weeks, start feeding at maximum of 0.0209 MJ/kg/day

Source: *BMJ 2008; 336 (7659): 1495–1498.* Reproduced with permission of BMJ Publishing Ltd.

**Figure 22.4** A NBM sign hanging by a patient's bed

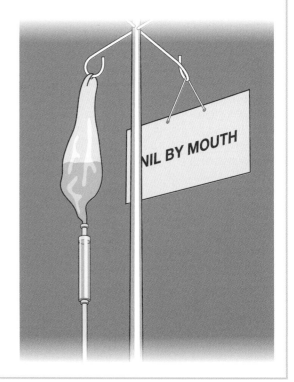

NIL BY MOUTH

*Medical School at a Glance*, First Edition. Rachel K. Thomas © 2017 John Wiley & Sons, Ltd. Published 2017 by John Wiley & Sons, Ltd.

Nutrition is a **complex field**, and is covered in varying degrees at different medical schools. Try to start thinking about the **nutritional status of a patient** as a medical student, even if the topic is only covered minimally during your formal studies. Nutrition has a **significant impact** on patients and their **recovery**. Their nutritional status can even be the **cause** for their hospital admission (Figure 22.1).

Patients' **attitudes** towards food are **multi-factorial** and complicated, and a **psychological overlay** to nutritional problems may also be present. Taking a thorough history is key in assessing nutrition, as there may be **physical reasons** for a patient's nutritional problems.

Numerous **factors** lead to **poor nutrition**:

- Impaired absorption (e.g. cystic fibrosis)
- Inadequate intake (e.g. anorexia nervosa)
- Increased intestinal losses (e.g. post-small bowel resection)
- Dietary restrictions (e.g. certain renal or liver diseases)
- Increased catabolic demand (e.g. cachectic states)
- Genetic disorders (e.g. Prader–Willi syndrome)
- Poor diet (e.g. leading to obesity).

## Assessing nutrition

Adequate assessment of nutrition requires:

- A detailed history (including drug and travel history)
- Examination
- Measurements (weight, height, BMI)
- Tests (most commonly, blood tests).

There are many **nutrition screening tools** like the subjective global assessment of nutritional status (http://img.medscapestatic.com/pi/meds/ckb/93/26893tn.jpg) or the mini-nutritional assessment (www.mna-elderly.com).

**Body mass index** (BMI) is often used to determine where a patient lies on a **standardised scale**. BMI is calculated by dividing the weight (in kg) by the height (in metres squared). **Dosage** for some medications requires knowledge of the patient's BMI or weight, for example paracetamol doses for children are based on their weight. Also examine the skin for signs of vitamin deficiency (e.g. angular chelitis). Does the patient look wasted or obese?

## Investigating nutritional status

**Blood tests** to assess nutritional status include tests for levels of **vitamins** and **minerals** in the blood (e.g. vitamin D, folic acid, calcium, magnesium, phosphate) and for the overall level of protein in the blood (e.g. albumin). Occasionally, other tests are required (e.g. DEXA scan), depending on the history and examination, to investigate further the cause or effect of nutritional deficiency.

## Managing nutritional deficits and over-nutrition

As a medical student try to spend time with **dietitians**. Patients with nutritional problems are referred to dietitians, who help manage nutritional deficiencies or over-nutrition (Figure 22.2).

Some patients require management through following **specific diets** (e.g. a gluten-free diet for coeliac disease; a low protein diet for renal failure). Other patients need **psychological, medical** (e.g. endocrine support) or **surgical** (e.g. bariatric surgery)

input. Guidelines have been established to target the management of specific conditions (e.g. anorexia nervosa and the MARSIPAN guidelines). The Royal College of Physicians have published the **Top Ten Tips** for various aspects of nutrition (https://www.rcplondon.ac.uk/projects/outputs/nutrition-top-ten-tips).

Nutritional support can be provided in several ways. Special nutritional drinks or supplements (e.g. Ensure™) can be used as **caloric supplements** for patients who have a low oral intake. **Vitamin supplements** (e.g. vitamin D or a multivitamin) can also be used when required.

## Enteral and total parenteral nutrition

Sometimes **enteral nutrition** (EN) or **total parenteral nutrition** (TPN) is required. This could be for physical (e.g. severe gastro-oesophageal reflux, oesophageal strictures or surgery) or for other reasons (e.g. anorexia nervosa, overnight feeding).

EN means that the patient receives food **directly** into their stomach. The 'food' received is frequently a specific form of **liquid nutrition** formulated according to the patient's requirements. EN can be achieved via either a **nasogastric** or an **orogastric tube,** to send the food directly from the nose or mouth or to the stomach, respectively. A **gastrostomy** (or percutaneous gastrostomy, PEG) or a **jejunostomy** takes food directly into the stomach or jejunum, respectively.

TPN is nutrition given through a **vein** and is used for patients who are unable to obtain sufficient nutrition from their gut. This could be for various reasons, such as extensive intra-abdominal surgery. TPN is a special formula of nutrition containing electrolytes, carbohydrates, fats (lipids), protein and trace elements.

EN is preferred to TPN because there are fewer complications (e.g. infection), it is cheaper, and it offers a better quality of life to the patient.

Also consider how to **re-introduce food** to patients who have been starved or on TPN for a long time. Patients can be at risk of re-feeding syndrome (Figure 22.3).

## Nil by mouth

As a medical student you may see patients who are **'nil by mouth'** (NBM) (Figure 22.4). NBM is usually stipulated to reduce the risk of **aspiration** of oral and gastric contents. (Breathing these contents into the lungs could result in complications such as infections including aspiration pneumonia, or death). NBM is required for various reasons:

- For a patient with reduced consciousness
- Before surgery/anaesthetic
- After surgery or anaesthetic
- For a patient with an unsafe swallow
- Conditions where resting the gut is indicated.

When you see the NBM sign, ensure that you do not accidentally give the patient anything to eat or drink.

## Protected meal times

Ensure that you do not interrupt patients during their meals. Most hospitals have **protected meal times**, so that patients can eat **undisturbed** – ensure that you respect this. You may be able to help some patients with their meals, after discussing if it would be appropriate with ward staff.

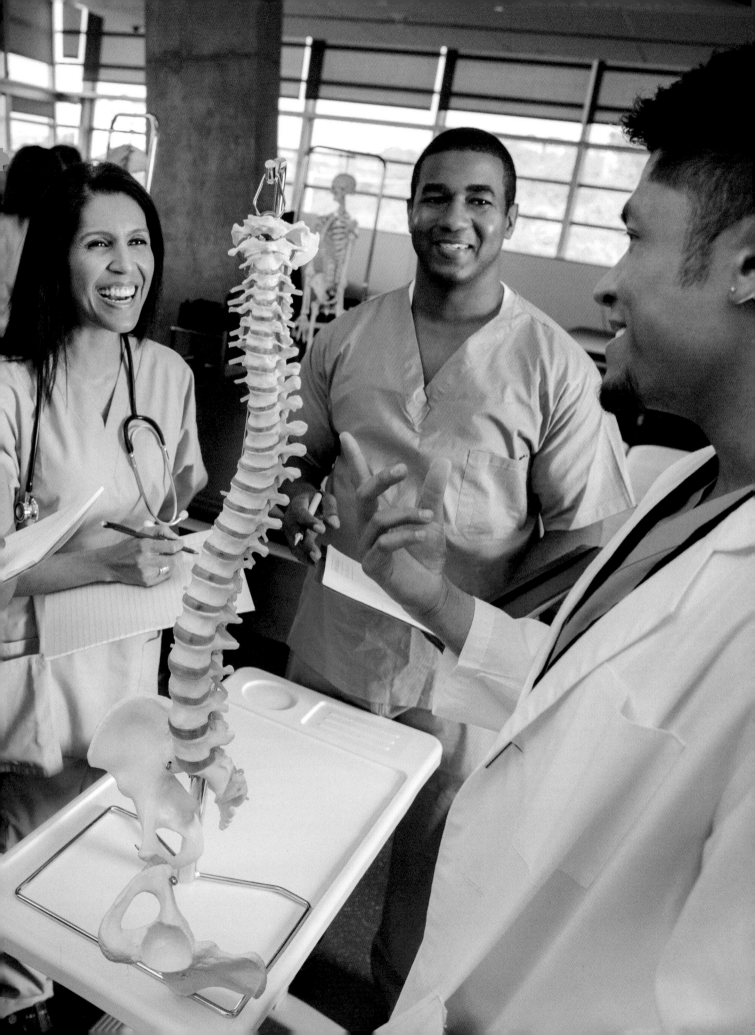

# Considering and managing a patient

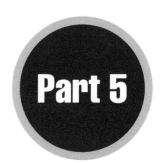

**Part 5**

## Chapters

# 23 Investigations

**Figure 23.1** Common non-invasive bedside tests – urine dipstick, ECG, peak flow and spirometry

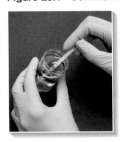
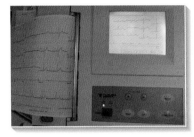
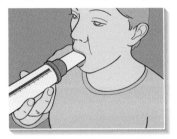
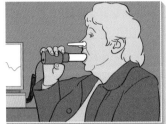

**Figure 23.2** Venepuncture to collect blood samples, and some different collection bottles

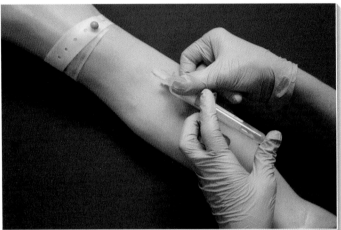
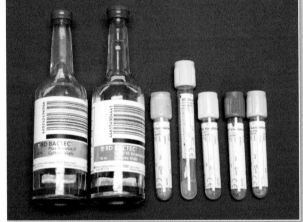

Source: Thomas R. Practical Medical Procedures at a Glance (2015). Reproduced with permission of John Wiley & Sons Ltd.

**Figure 23.3** Common types of medical imaging – X-ray, ultrasound, MRI, and CT

| X-ray | Ultrasound | MRI | CT |
| --- | --- | --- | --- |

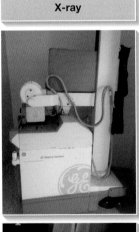
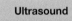
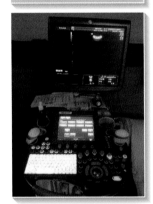
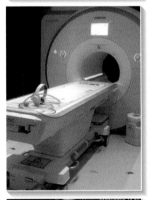
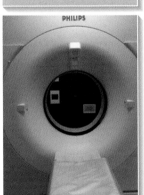
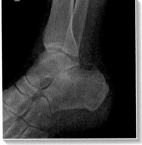
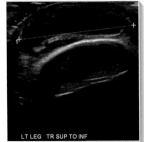
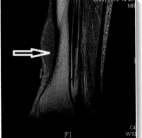
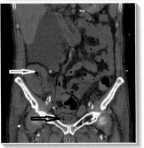

Source: Gleadle J. et al. Clinical Investigations at a Glance (2017). Reproduced with permission of John Wiley & Sons Ltd.

*Medical School at a Glance*, First Edition. Rachel K. Thomas © 2017 John Wiley & Sons, Ltd. Published 2017 by John Wiley & Sons, Ltd.

# What are investigations?

**Investigations** are used to help determine the patient's diagnosis, and how effective their treatment is.

They can be **non-invasive,** such as a urine dip measurement, or **invasive,** such as venepuncture (blood tests). They can also be divided up into **bedside tests, imaging** and **laboratory tests.**

Become **comfortable** with these investigations at medical school, as they are one of your **tools** to help you figure out how to treat your patients once you become a doctor. Requesting investigations correctly and appropriately, interpreting the results and then acting efficiently and suitably on the results is key. As with all procedures, the patient needs to be informed of the risks and benefits of an investigation, along with the implications of the **investigation's results,** and give their **consent.** There will be **guidelines** for the appropriate use of investigations for each area you are based in, so ensure that you are aware of, and adhere to, all **local and national guidelines.** These guidelines are designed not only for **patient safety,** but also for **appropriate resource allocation.**

Investigations need to be requested on **specific forms,** which may be online or on paper, depending on **local protocols.** Usually, a **specific question** will need to be formulated as to why the investigation is required. Remember that the questions are read, and so a 'please' and a 'thank you' may help speed the process along! It is key to understand that, as a doctor, once you have requested an investigation, it is your **responsibility** to ensure that its results are **checked** and **acted upon.** It is also your responsibility to ensure that samples are **labelled clearly** and **correctly,** and that they are sent to the **appropriate area** for testing. In cases where **urgent** results are required, it may expedite the process if the department receiving the sample is telephoned and forewarned to expect it.

# Bedside tests

Bedside tests are literally those that can be carried out at the side of the patient's bed (Figure 23.1). These are simple tests, such as:

- Urinalysis
- Electrocardiogram (ECG)
- Peak flow measurement
- Spirometry.

# Laboratory tests

These tests are performed on a sample of fluid or tissue that must be carefully labelled and sent off to a laboratory for analysis (Figure 23.2).

## 1 Biochemical

- *Electrolytes:* commonly, potassium ($K^+$), sodium ($Na^+$) and also calcium ($Ca^{2+}$), phosphate ($PO_4^{3-}$), magnesium ($Mg^+$) and chloride ($Cl^-$)
- *Renal function:* urea, creatinine
- *Liver function:* albumin, alanine aminotransferase (ALT), aspartate transaminase (AST), alkaline phosphatase (ALP)
- Blood glucose

- *Cardiac enzymes:* troponin T, lactate dehydrogenase (LDH), creatinine kinase (CK)
- Amylase.

Urea and electrolytes measurements are commonly referred to as U&Es.

## 2 Haematological

- *Full blood count* (FBC): haemoglobin (Hb), white cell count (WCC), platelets
- Clotting or coagulation studies
- Inflammatory markers, such as C-reactive protein (CRP, and erythrocyte sedimentation rate (ESR).

## 3 Pathological

- *Microbiology:* microscopy, culture and sensitivity (MC&S), blood cultures
- *Histology:* tissue biopsies
- *Cytology:* cell samples
- Post-mortem examinations (PM).

# Imaging

Imaging generally requires more advanced **specialist equipment** and **detailed interpretation** (Figure 23.3). These tests provide a **visual representation** of an area of the body, which can then be carefully inspected for any abnormalities:

- Plain film radiographs, or X-rays
- Ultrasound
- Computed tomography (CT)
- Magnetic resonance imaging (MRI).

There are some common, acceptable abbreviations that are used for X-rays –chest X-ray is CXR, and abdominal X-ray is AXR.

Many of the imaging investigations can be observed by visiting the **Radiography department.** Seeing the various scans being taken can help greatly with learning about them. Seeing the patient and understanding their presenting signs and symptoms can also help with learning to read images, which at first you may think are abstract hazes of black, grey and white!

**Hints and Tips:**

- Ensure you are familiar with **local** and **national protocols** and **guidelines** for requesting tests
- Ensure that you become **comfortable** with the different investigations, including explaining how they are performed to a patient, during medical school

**Did you know?**

Aspects of imaging can be dangerous:
- Imaging such as X-rays and CT scans use **radiation**
- MRIs have **strong magnetic fields** and cannot be used with certain implanted devices
- Contrast administered intravenously can cause **allergic** reactions

You must be able to **justify** exposing a patient to these risks, and ensure that the patient is **aware** of them prior to the procedure.

# 24 Considering diagnoses

**Figure 24.1** Test and treatment thresholds in the diagnostic process

Test threshold

Treatment threshold

0%

100%

**Probability of diagnosis**

No testing required
when probability is
below test threshold

Testing required when
probability lies between
test and treatment thresholds

Testing complete and
treatment begins when
probability is above
treatment threshold

*Source: Richardson et al., 2002. The Process of Diagnosis. The American Medical Association.*

**Figure 24.2** Some possible causes of chest pain

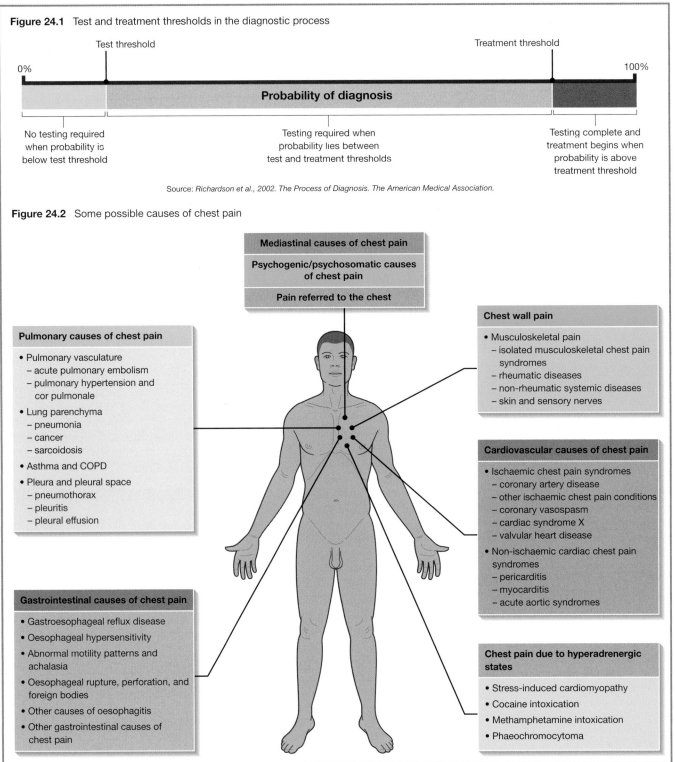

**Mediastinal causes of chest pain**

**Psychogenic/psychosomatic causes
of chest pain**

**Pain referred to the chest**

**Chest wall pain**

- Musculoskeletal pain
  - isolated musculoskeletal chest pain
    syndromes
  - rheumatic diseases
  - non-rheumatic systemic diseases
  - skin and sensory nerves

**Pulmonary causes of chest pain**

- Pulmonary vasculature
  - acute pulmonary embolism
  - pulmonary hypertension and
    cor pulmonale
- Lung parenchyma
  - pneumonia
  - cancer
  - sarcoidosis
- Asthma and COPD
- Pleura and pleural space
  - pneumothorax
  - pleuritis
  - pleural effusion

**Cardiovascular causes of chest pain**

- Ischaemic chest pain syndromes
  - coronary artery disease
  - other ischaemic chest pain conditions
  - coronary vasospasm
  - cardiac syndrome X
  - valvular heart disease
- Non-ischaemic cardiac chest pain
  syndromes
  - pericarditis
  - myocarditis
  - acute aortic syndromes

**Gastrointestinal causes of chest pain**

- Gastroesophageal reflux disease
- Oesophageal hypersensitivity
- Abnormal motility patterns and
  achalasia
- Oesophageal rupture, perforation, and
  foreign bodies
- Other causes of oesophagitis
- Other gastrointestinal causes of
  chest pain

**Chest pain due to hyperadrenergic
states**

- Stress-induced cardiomyopathy
- Cocaine intoxication
- Methamphetamine intoxication
- Phaeochromocytoma

The importance of determining the **correct diagnosis** for a patient is obvious. There are various methods to help you start considering diagnoses. Having a **framework** of diagnoses can be helpful, not only at the beginning of your medical studies, but throughout your career as a doctor. It is important to also consider **other possible diagnoses** even if a particular one seems **obvious** to you (often referred to as a 'barn door' if it is very obvious or typical), as this will help ensure that you consider **atypical presentations** or other **life-threatening conditions** that could be catastrophic if they were missed.

## What are differential diagnoses?

**Differential diagnoses** are basically a list of **possible causes** for why the patient is unwell. Each is a diagnosis that **reasonably** fits the presentation of signs and symptoms. (Remember that **signs** are things that you **observe**, while **symptoms** are things that the **patient reports** – sym'p'toms and 'p'atient both have a 'p' in them to help you to remember that symptoms are something the patient reports.)

It is very important to include **less likely**, but **more dangerous**, conditions on this list, as these are the conditions that you will need to rule out first. It is also important to ensure that you have included all the **common causes**.

The possible causes are considered against each other, investigations are carried out and the most likely condition or conditions identified are then **treated** following a **management plan** (Figure 24.1).

## Formulating differential diagnoses

A useful way of formulating a differential diagnosis can be to use the concept of a **surgical sieve**. This can help ensure you do not miss out any causes. This is a commonly used technique, and can be especially useful in **oral examinations** when you may be nervous and forgetful (see Chapter 32). It is a method of ordering your thoughts, when asked about the causes of a condition, to give an answer with **structure**. It can also be a useful tool for helping to explain the possible causes of symptoms and signs to a patient, before you have received the results from investigations.

A **common surgical sieve** is broken into the following groups:
- Congenital
- Acquired
  - Vascular
  - Infective, idiopathic
  - Trauma, tumour
  - Autoimmune
  - Metabolic, mental
  - Inflammatory
  - Neurological
  - Degenerative
  - Environmental, endocrine
  - Functional.

The acquired causes can be remembered by a mnemonic such as 'VITAMIN DEF'.

Often, differential diagnoses can be based on the anatomy in the relevant area, then causes for the condition within this anatomical structure are defined (Figure 24.2).

Diagnosis is often abbreviated to Dx, and differential diagnosis DDx or $\Delta\Delta$.

To create a differential, consider a full list of possible conditions fitting the clinical picture and the patient history, ensuring that you include **atypical presentations** and **life-threatening conditions** – even if you think that they are relatively unlikely.

Then consider the probability or likelihood of each condition, by factoring in any extra available information to increase or decrease the chance of each diagnosis.

Factor in information from the **history** (Was there a recent operation or illness? Have they recently been travelling?), the **examination** (Is there any calf swelling? Are there extra heart sounds?) and **investigations** (Does a CXR show consolidation? Is the ECG normal?).

The most likely cause for the condition is then referred to as a **working diagnosis**.

It is advisable to keep considering other likely or life-threatening diagnoses, often referred to as **active alternate diagnoses**.

## Diagnostic criteria

**Diagnostic criteria** assist you to formulate a diagnosis.

These are usually **several specific symptoms, signs** and **investigation results** that fit pre-defined aspects for a disease presentation.

Specific diagnostic criteria are readily available from sites such as the American College of Rheumatology (ACR) for rheumatological conditions such as rheumatoid arthritis, or the *Diagnostic and Statistical Manual of Mental Disorders*, 5th edition (DSM-5), for psychiatric conditions such as autism.

## Pattern recognition

As they become more experienced, some clinicians start to use **pattern recognition** for common presentations of certain diseases. In doing this, they merge pattern recognition with experience and logic, but to be able to do this they need to have seen many cases of many illnesses. While you are learning, it is advisable to think of differential diagnoses in a framework or structured way, even when one disease seems very obvious, to ensure that you are not missing anything. This can help minimise the chances of **misdiagnosis**, which could obviously have fatal consequences.

**Hints and Tips:**
- Consider **life-threatening conditions** in your differential diagnosis
- Use a **framework** to ensure that all causes are considered
- Familiarise yourself with the different **diagnostic criteria**

# 25 Presenting a patient

**Figure 25.1** Presenting a history and examination

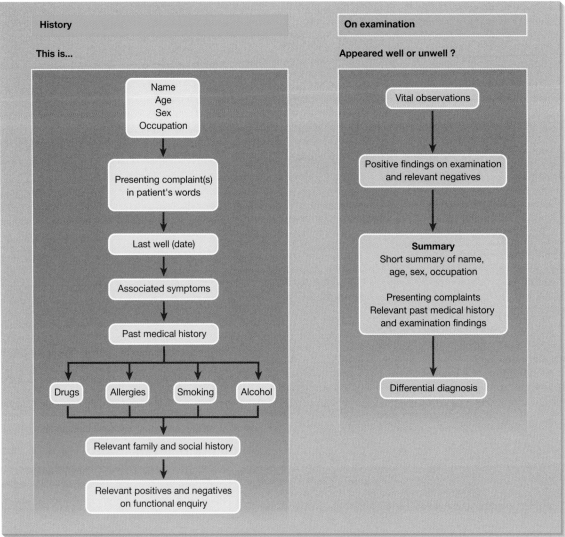

| History | On examination |
| --- | --- |
| **This is...** | **Appeared well or unwell ?** |

History flow:
- Name / Age / Sex / Occupation
- Presenting complaint(s) in patient's words
- Last well (date)
- Associated symptoms
- Past medical history
  - Drugs
  - Allergies
  - Smoking
  - Alcohol
- Relevant family and social history
- Relevant positives and negatives on functional enquiry

On examination flow:
- Vital observations
- Positive findings on examination and relevant negatives
- **Summary**
  Short summary of name, age, sex, occupation

  Presenting complaints
  Relevant past medical history and examination findings
- Differential diagnosis

Source: *Gleadle J. History and Clinical Examination at a Glance, 3rd edn (2012). Reproduced with permission of John Wiley & Sons Ltd.*

**Figure 25.2** Presenting a patient's image

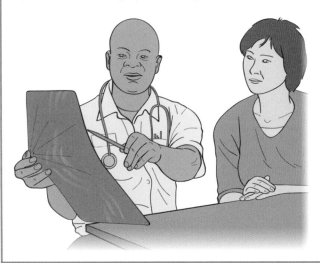

**Hints and Tips:**
When describing the image, different areas on:
- X-rays are **radio-dense**
- USSs are **echogenic**
- MRIs have **signal intensity**
- CT have **attenuation**

*Medical School at a Glance*, First Edition. Rachel K. Thomas © 2017 John Wiley & Sons, Ltd. Published 2017 by John Wiley & Sons, Ltd.

**P**resenting a patient is when you speak about a patient to convey key information about them to other clinicians or healthcare professionals.

Like anything new, **presenting** a patient can be challenging the first few times you do it. Start **practising** this as soon as you can, and, like many other areas of medicine, it will become the **important tool** that it is, rather than a difficulty.

When presenting a **history**, speak **clearly** and **confidently**. Start with the patient's name, age and reason for presenting to hospital (Figure 25.1).

For example: 'This is Mr Clark, a 38-year-old man with a 2-day history of lower back pain.'

For pain, characterise the pain fully, such as 'it is in his central lumbar region, and came on suddenly. It is of a burning nature, and radiates down his left leg. Lying down and simple analgesia have helped his pain, and walking makes it worse. It is worse at the end of the day, and is, at worst, a 7/10 severity.'

After this, proceed to outline the other areas of the patient history, such as the past medical history, drug history, allergies, family history and social history (see Chapter 19).

When presenting a patient, include **important negatives** as well as the **important positives**, as you are trying to rule in and rule out various conditions as you present.

After presenting what the patient has told you, move on to presenting the findings in examination, investigations, results and a management plan for your suspected differential diagnoses.

Determining what to say and what not to say in a presentation of a patient takes **time** and **experience**. There is often a **time pressure**, as the clinician you are speaking with may be very busy, but it is better to say too much than not enough. When you are learning, ensure you **cover everything** so that you do not miss out important facts.

**Hints and Tips:**
- **Following** a patient, from taking their history to their having imaging, and then trying to interpret this imaging can greatly help your learning
- Always check and state the **patient's details** when presenting

## Presenting images

When a patient has an **investigation** performed, such as an X-ray, it is the responsibility of the requesting doctor to ensure that the image or results are **reviewed**. There are usually **radiologists** available to interpret images; however, this will not always be the case. You should develop a **system** early on in medical school for reading, interpreting and presenting images (Figure 25.2). Developing a system or **framework** for this helps ensure that you do not miss anything. It can help you look at the bigger picture first, and then applying your system to find details. This approach is particularly helpful when you are tired, as you doubtlessly will be as a junior doctor and on your first twilight or night shifts, or nervous – as you may be during examinations or with a new consultant.

Practise looking at the **actual images** before looking at their **formal reports**. This way you can learn as you go, and **self-test** to see what you noticed and what you missed. It can be tempting, particularly in the beginning, to feel overwhelmed and go straight for the report. You need to see quite a few images before you can spot differences between some types of images. Going with a patient to see the images being taken is time well spent (see Chapter 23). Remember that images are clues to help you figure out the best treatment for a patient – so ensure you consider their **overall clinical picture**.

When presenting, start with the **obvious details** – these are **key** (and they can also buy you time to think about what to say next). The obvious details are included on the image, and can be read out – the patient's **name**, date of birth (calculate the **age**), the **type** and **anatomical location** of the image (X-ray, MRI, ultrasound, CT of the abdomen) and the **date** it was taken on. Always check the **patient's details** before you begin, as reading the wrong patient's information does not help anyone – and can indeed cause great harm if this information is acted upon.

Comment on any **obvious abnormalities**. It can be helpful to take a **'step back'**, and look at the image as a whole, to see if there are any areas that 'look wrong'. Comment on the presence of any **medical devices** (such as ECG leads, implantable defibrillators, nasogastric tubes, surgical closure clips, ventilation equipment). You do not need to say why they are there, just comment that they are there, and use this to help build up a picture of what is going on with the patient. Remember, in much the same vein as if you have not documented something, it has not happened, if you do not comment on it, it is not there (and remember this especially in an exam setting). As you become more proficient at reading images, you will learn what to comment on and what to leave out, but at first, and particularly during exams, comment on it all!

It can take time to develop a **suitable system** for interpreting images that works for you. A suggested system involves looking at each part of the **anatomy** for any abnormalities. This needs to be carried out in a systematic way, so that you do not miss anything or become distracted when you find an abnormality, as there may be more than one.

# 26 Consent and capacity

**Figure 26.1** A patient may give actions that imply consent

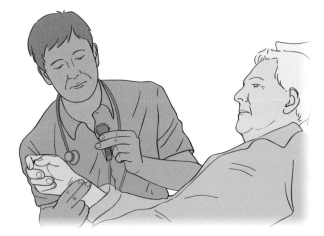

**Figure 26.3** The Mental Capacity Act

**Gives any adult with capacity the right to make:**
- Advance decision(s)
- Lasting Power of Attorney

**And**

Says how to decide if someone has capacity

**And**

**For any adult without capacity it tells professionals to:**
- Act in their best interests
- Consult family/friends about decisions
- Appoint IMCA for important decisions
- Apply Deprivation of Liberty Safeguards (DoLS) to anyone deprived of liberty

Source: *Katona C. et al. Psychiatry at a Glance, 5th edn (2012). Reproduced with permission of John Wiley & Sons Ltd.*

**Box 26.1** The Mental Capacity Act says

- Everyone has the right to make his or her own decisions. Health and care professionals should always assume an individual has the capacity to make a decision themselves, unless it is proved otherwise through a capacity assessment
- Individuals must be given help to make a decision themselves. This might include, e.g. providing the person with information in a format that is easier for them to understand
- Just because someone makes what those caring for them consider to be an 'unwise' decision, they should not be treated as lacking the capacity to make that decision. Everyone has the right to make their own life choices, where they have the capacity to do so
- Where someone is judged not to have the capacity to make a specific decision (following a capacity assessment), that decision can be taken for them, but it must be in their best interests
- Treatment and care provided to someone who lacks capacity should be the least restrictive of their basic rights and freedoms possible, while still providing the required treatment and care

Source: *http://www.nhs.uk/conditions/social-care-and-support-guide/pages/mental-capacity.aspx*

**Figure 26.2** Some procedures need formal, written, informed consent

**Patient identifier/label**

**Name of proposed procedure or course of treatment** (include brief explanation if medical term not clear) .........................................................
..................................................................................................................

**Statement of health professional** (to be filled in by health professional with appropriate knowledge of proposed procedure, as specified in consent policy)

I have explained the procedure to the patient. In particular, I have explained:

The intended benefits .............................................................................
..................................................................................................................
..................................................................................................................

Serious or frequently occurring risks ....................................................
..................................................................................................................
..................................................................................................................

Any extra procedures which may become necessary during the procedure

☐ Blood transfusion ...............................................................................

☐ Other procedure (please specify) .......................................................
..................................................................................................................

I have also discussed what the procedure is likely to involve, the benefits and risks of any available alternative treatments (including no treatment) and any particular concerns of this patient.

## Hints and Tips:

To give valid **consent**, a patient must:
- Have **capacity**
- Act **voluntarily**

To have capacity, a patient must:
- **Understand** the information
- **Retain** the information
- **Weigh** the information's implications
- **Communicate** a decision

## Did you know?

Patients may lack capacity due to many causes, including:
- Brain injury
- Stroke
- Dementia
- Mental health issues

*Medical School at a Glance*, First Edition. Rachel K. Thomas © 2017 John Wiley & Sons, Ltd. Published 2017 by John Wiley & Sons, Ltd.

# Consent

**Consent** is a **valid permission** that you must **legally gain** prior to any **intervention** on a patient. An intervention is roughly defined as something that could **change an outcome** for, or **impact** on, a patient. According to the GMC, consent must be obtained before:
- Treating a patient
- Carrying out an investigation on a patient
- Involving a patient in a screening process
- Including a patient in teaching
- Including a patient in research.

All of these activities involve various **decisions** made between the patient and you or their doctor. As a medical student, you will need to gain consent from patients prior to your interactions with them. Even seemingly **simple, non-invasive procedures and processes**, such as taking a blood pressure or history, need to be consented for.

In some cases, a patient's **action** can give **implied consent**. For instance, a patient may offer their arm for you to take their pulse (Figure 26.1). In other cases, such as for surgical procedures, consent must be gained **formally** and recorded in **writing** (usually on a consent form; Figure 26.2).

It is better to ask specifically for consent and to gain senior input to help with this, particularly if you are unsure. As a medical student, you will not generally be required to determine capacity or gain consent without senior input.

Consent needs to be **informed**. This means that the **risks** and **benefits** of an intervention need to be explained and understood by the patient. The **reason** for the intervention, and **how** the intervention will be carried out, and **what could happen** if it does not occur needs to be explained. Therefore you **cannot gain consent for a procedure that you are not able to do yourself.**

Consent is only valid if it is given:
- Voluntarily
- With capacity.

Consent can be **withdrawn** at a later date, provided that the patient still has capacity to do so. Patients also have the right to **refuse** an intervention, treatment or activity, provided that they have capacity, and they have made the decision voluntarily. Part of gaining consent is ensuring that a patient is aware of this right.

If you approach a patient and would like to take a history from them, you could ask something along the lines of:

'Hi, my name is Rachel Thomas, and I am a final year medical student. Are you happy to speak with me today? I'd like to ask you some questions about why you are in hospital. It is purely for my learning, and won't affect your treatment, so you don't have to speak with me if you don't feel like it.'

If a patient **declines** to give consent and does not wish to speak with you, **thank them** and **respect their wishes**.

Once a patient has reached their decision, provided it was made voluntarily and they have capacity, you must **respect** and **adhere** to this, even if you disagree with it. For difficult situations, such as living organ donation, life-saving treatment refusal and treating minors, advice and decision-making can be esca-lated up through various levels of seniority – eventually even up to the **High Court**.

# Capacity

**Capacity** is addressed in the Mental Capacity Act 2005, which came into effect in the UK in 2007 (Figure 26.3; Box 26.1). Capacity is the ability for a patient to:
1 **Understand** the information that they are given
2 **Retain** the information that they are given
3 **Weigh** this information 'in the balance', such that they are able to look at the pros and cons of various outcomes
4 **Communicate** a decision, based on this information.

All four of these aspects need to be present for a doctor to **legally** be able to perform an **intervention** on a patient. The communication of the decision does not necessarily have to be of a specified format, if this is not possible for the patient. For instance, if a patient cannot speak, they can write the decision instead.

As a patient can **refuse treatments**, provided they have capacity, treating a patient against their will is a prosecutable offence called **battery**. Always check with a senior if you are unsure in any case. There is guidance available from many sources, including the GMC, for determining and learning about capacity.

Generally, it is assumed that someone **over the age of 16** has capacity unless it is established that they do not. **All efforts** must be made to help them make a decision by enhancing and enabling their abilities, and someone cannot be deemed as lacking capacity until this has been done. The above four aspects need to have been formally evaluated and documented in the notes in some cases.

Patients **under the age of 16** are assumed to not have capacity – however, in some cases, they may be deemed to have **Fraser** or **Gillick competence**, named after a case in the House of Lords in 1985. If a child is not Gillick competent, then those with **parental responsibility** authorise the child's treatment on their behalf. This is usually the child's parent, but not always. If a child is **Fraser or Gillick competent,** then **parental consent is not required**.

If the child will suffer without a treatment and the parental responsibility consent cannot be gained, then a **court decision** can be applied for. Treatments must be carried out the in the **best interests** of the child in an emergency.

The areas of consent and capacity can be complex and confusing, so never assume, and always seek **senior or specialist input.** Discussing these areas with the **psychiatry team** can also help with your learning in difficult cases, particularly if you are unclear as to why or how a decision was made.

### Did you know?

**Lord Fraser** was the judge in the landmark competence case in 1985 in which Mrs Gillick challenged a doctor for prescribing contraception for her daughter, who was under 16, without her parental consent. In this case, it was decided that the daughter's mental or physical health would suffer if she did not receive the contraceptive treatment and advice, and that to give it to her was in her best interests – regardless of the lack of parental consent.

# 27 Breaking bad news

**Figure 27.1** A guide for clinical staff in breaking bad news

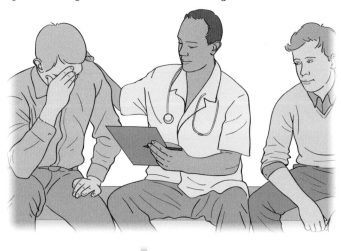

**Figure 27.2** The SPIKES protocol

Consultation with relatives present. **SPIKES** is a six-step protocol which has been shown to improve the confidence of clinicans who use it when breaking bad news to cancer patients:

- **S**etting up the interview
- Assessing the patient's **P**erception
- Obtaining the patient's **I**nvitation, as shunning information is a valid psychological coping mechanism
- Giving **K**nowledge and information to the patient
- Addressing the patient's **E**motions with **E**mpathetic response
- Having a **S**trategy and **S**ummarising

Source: *Baile W, et al. (2000) SPIKES- A Six Step Protocol for Delivering Bad News: Application to the Patient with Cancer. The Oncologist 5:302-311.*

**Prepare yourself**

- Check the patient's history, results and management
- Rehearse the interview mentally
- Think about questions and answers
- Think about who else in the team could be helpful – such as a specialist nurse or family member

**Prepare the setting**

- Privacy and take your time
- Sit and keep eye contact with the patient
- Minimise interruptions such as from your bleep or mobile – give it to someone on your team

**Prepare the patient**

- Determine what the patient knows already
- Determine how much the patient wishes to know

**Provide information**

- Use appropriate language – non-technical, no jargon
- Deliver news at a pace the patient can handle, in small 'chunks' of information
- Break the news gently but clearly, avoiding euphemisms
- Give the patient time for questions

**After the news**

- Record what was said, and who it was said to – including the terms you used, and the plans that were made
- Discuss with other members of the healtchcare team – including the GP and MDT

**Provide a plan**

- Provide a plan with treatments and management – even if few options are available, such as pain control
- Plan to meet with family if the patient would like this

**Provide support**

- Ask the patient how they are feeling
- Convey empathy with phrases such as "I can imagine how you might be feeling"
- Give the patient time to talk about how they are feeling
- Listen

Source: *Based upon National Council for Hospice and Specialist Palliative Care Services (http://www.cen.scot.nhs.uk/files/4b-breaking_bad_news-ireland.pdf).*

While **bad news** can mean different things depending on the context and to whom it is delivered, it generally relates to a message that points to a **very different future** for those involved. It can mean delivering news that a treatment has been unsuccessful, a further procedure is required, a malignancy has been detected or someone has died.

The importance of **good communication skills** is highlighted when bad news has to be delivered. Communication is a basic skill that needs to be **practised** while you are in medical school, and so does the delivery of bad news (Figure 27.1). There has been an increased focus in recent years on this aspect of medicine, as a poor 'bedside manner' is no longer acceptable, and on the requisite verbal and non-verbal communication skills (see Chapter 9).

As with any skills, you need to **watch** them in action in order to learn them. This is also the case in the breaking of bad news. Ensure that the doctor, patient and family do not mind you being present while this difficult conversation is occurring. It may be more appropriate for the doctor who is about to deliver the news to ask the patient or family if they mind you being present in your absence. If they do mind, obviously this needs to be respected, and if necessary you can discuss the situation later with the doctor in question.

There are various protocols and pathways that have been developed to assist in the delivery of bad news, such as the BREAKS protocol, the Calgary–Cambridge framework and the SPIKES protocol (Figure 27.2). Reading these can be of great assistance to your learning of this skill.

As a medical student, you may be in a unique position to **help** the patient and their family or carer. Because of clinical demands and time constraints, doctors may not have the time to spend with the patient after the delivery of bad news. However, if the doctor, patient, family or carers request it, you, as a student, can offer a presence or comfort that other medical professionals may simply not have the time for. Determining this is a sensitive skill. In some situations, asking if there is anything you can do after the news has been broken is appropriate.

## Key steps in breaking bad news

As a medical student, you will not generally be required to break bad news to patients, but will most likely be asked to do so in exams. However, it is important to start thinking about this challenging area, and developing ways to deliver this news when you are a junior doctor.

First, you will need to ensure that you hold the conversation in as **private** a place as possible, where you will not be disturbed.

As with other communication, **introduce yourself** prior to delivery of any news and ensure you use **clear, jargon-free language**.

When you begin, determine how much the patient and their family or carer already **know**, and check they **understand** what you are saying as the conversation progresses.

If a **translator** is required, it is preferable to speak with them prior to their conversation with the patient, family or carer, so they are also prepared, enabling the delivery of the bad news to be as optimal as possible.

Preparing the patient for the news with a 'warning shot', by using phrases such as 'I'm sorry but I've some bad news for you', can help to soften the impact of surprise somewhat. Also determine the particular **level of information** the patient would prefer, through asking them questions such as 'Would you like just a general overview, or specific information?'

**Questions** should be answered **directly** and clearly, yet **compassionately.** You should ensure that you give the patient, and their family or carer, time to ask questions during the conversation.

## After the delivery of bad news

The conversation relating to the breaking of bad news should be **documented** in the patient's notes. It is key to include **who** was spoken to, **what** was explained and any **follow-up plans** that were discussed.

Witnessing the breaking of bad news or breaking it yourself, can be **upsetting**. Ensure that you receive any **support** you need at these challenging times. While it can be tempting to dismiss the effect it can have on you, try to acknowledge and deal with it in a constructive way (see Chapter 5). It can also similarly affect the doctor delivering the news, and so speaking about it together can help you both.

Remember that **confidentiality** must be maintained and respected in any conversations. This includes discussions for personal support, as well as disclosure of a patient's condition and information with their family. Do not ever assume that the patient wants their family or carer to know everything that they, themselves, wish to know.

After the delivery of the news, pause to **reflect** on how this was done – reflection can help **improve** the process for next time, as there will indeed be a next time.

**Hints and Tips:**
- Observe the **communication skills** used in the delivery of bad news where possible
- **Respect the patient's wishes** if they do not wish you to be present when bad news is broken to them
- Offer to **sit** with the patient afterwards, if this is appropriate
- **Discuss sensitive areas** with your senior doctor or tutor
- **Seek support** for yourself if you feel you need it

# 28 Prescribing

**Figure 28.1** Acceptable abbreviations for prescriptions

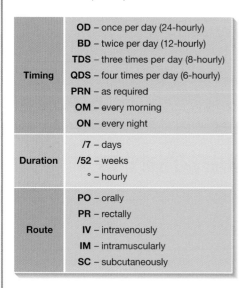

**Figure 28.2** Flow chart of electronic prescribing systems (EPS)

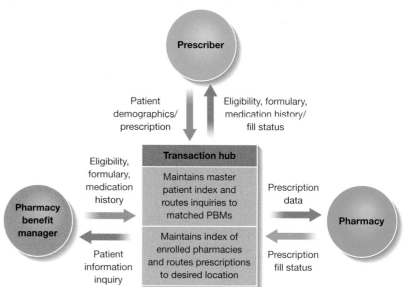

**Figure 28.3** Clearly cross out cards for practice

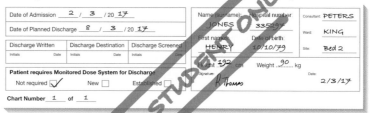

Source: *Thomas R. Practical Medical Procedures at a Glance (2015). Reproduced with permission of John Wiley & Sons Ltd.*

**Figure 28.4** Yellow-card reporting system for adverse effects

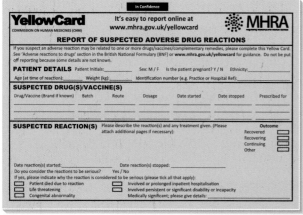

Source: *Reproduced with permission from the Medicines and Healthcare Products Regulatory Agency (MHRA).*

**Hints and Tips:**
- Remember to only use **acceptable abbreviations** when prescribing
- Spend time with patients **discussing** their medications, as this can help learn indications and side effects
- Always check patient **allergies** first!

# Learning to prescribe

Obviously, as a medical student, you are **not legally allowed** to prescribe medications. However, as a **junior doctor**, you will be prescribing medications frequently from your first day on the job, and so it is important to become comfortable with the process while still at medical school.

When learning about medications, it can be useful to start with **indications**, **contraindications, interactions** and **side effects** of medications, and then progress to **doses** and **administration routes**.

There are **acceptable abbreviations** for prescribing (Figure 28.1). However, some abbreviations are not acceptable. For instance, do not use μ for micro or u for units, but write the word out in whole, to avoid **errors** and **confusion**.

Talking with **pharmacists** and **specialist nurses** can help you learn about medications and their prescription. Speaking with **patients,** particularly about their experiences and side effects of various medications, can also be of great educational value. For instance, it is easier to remember that a patient needs to sit upright for 30–60 minutes after taking bisphosphonates if a patient has actually told you this. You can also help your team, and possibly ascertain issues around **compliance**, by spending time talking with a patient when the more senior doctors may not have the time to do so. For instance, a patient may reveal that they have backache when sitting for more than a few minutes, possibly indicating they are not taking their bisphosphonates correctly.

When learning about medications and their prescription, do so with a **questioning mind**. Ask yourself **why** medications are prescribed, why patients are taking their regular medications, are those medications required and are more medications in a given situation actually the 'right' approach? **Drug interactions** and **poly-pharmacy** (multiple medications) contribute a considerable burden for both the patient and the healthcare system.

# Electronic prescription systems

Prescriptions are written in different ways depending on the Healthcare Trust. Many prescriptions are now digital, with **e-prescribing** on **electronic prescribing systems** (EPS; Figure 28.2). Clinicians have an **independent login** and this acts as their 'signature' for the prescription. These systems offer benefits, such as:
- *Efficiency*: automatic and direct delivery to the pharmacy, many access points for delivery by nursing staff
- *Controls*: for errors and interactions
- *Safety*: no missing drug cards, no re-writing of old drug cards, no indecipherable handwriting, no bodyweight calculations for doses
- *Cost*: generic substitutes can automatically be suggested at a cheaper cost.

There are additional costs, both for software and clinician training, which have contributed to some Trusts not yet adopting EPS.

# Paper prescriptions

Many hospitals still use **paper medication prescription cards.** These are useful when learning prescribing. You can use spare cards to familiarise yourself with how to prescribe medications. Ensure that you clearly write 'Medical Student Practice' and block cross out the front of the card clearly, so that it is not mistaken for an actual patient's drug card (Figure 28.3). When being examined on prescribing, most medical schools use paper prescription cards, so it is advisable to become familiar with them.

On the different clinical rotations in different hospitals, familiarise yourself with each new type of medication card, as these tend to vary in different Healthcare Trusts.

When learning to prescribe, ensure that you develop good habits. Ensure that the prescription is **legible, neat**, and written in block **capitals**.

Before prescribing anything, ascertain if the patient has any **allergies.** Most cards have a section on the front of the drug card for this to be documented – and this can be recorded as 'no known drug allergies' (NKDA) if this is the case. It is also good practice to ask about any homeopathic, over-the-counter (OTC) or naturopathic medications that the patient is taking.

You also need to consider **interactions** and whether any **co-morbidities** (such as liver or renal failure) are present before prescribing medications, as these can alter the doses (and sometimes the medications) that are required.

# Safe prescriptions

Always check doses in the *British National Formulary* (BNF). Throughout your career you will need to keep this handy, but particularly when learning to prescribe. The BNF also has a **Yellow Card** system, which is used for reporting any suspected **adverse drug reactions**. It is a removable piece of yellow paper that is included in the back of the book, which the clinician fills in and posts without charge to the **Medicines and Healthcare Products Regulatory Agency** (MHRA; Figure 28.4).

Always check **local protocols** and **guidelines**, as certain areas have different microbial sensitivities or available medications. Many hospitals have **microbial guidelines,** some of which can be downloaded as an app.

Resources such as the **National Institute For Health and Care Excellence** (NICE) provide treatment guidelines to help with your learning.

# Drug rounds

**Drugs rounds** are the time when medications are handed out to the patients on a ward, and they happen frequently every day and night. Ask nursing staff if you can join them on these rounds. Helping on a round can provide a means for you to contribute to the smooth running of the ward, and also facilitate your learning.

Patients often describe what their medication actually looks like, rather than the name and what the dose is. By attending a drug round, you can see the **colours** and **shapes** of the medications, and also learn '**real world**' information about them. For instance, some patients find certain pills difficult to swallow because of their size.

Remember that drug rounds are a **key mechanism** in the delivery of quality care, and **do not interrupt** the nurse in charge of dispensing medications if you are not actually helping her. Ensure that you ask in advance of joining a round, rather than approaching when one is already underway (see Chapter 13).

# 29 Documentation

**Figure 29.1** Ward rounds integrate aspects of the patient's care, and need to be carefully recorded

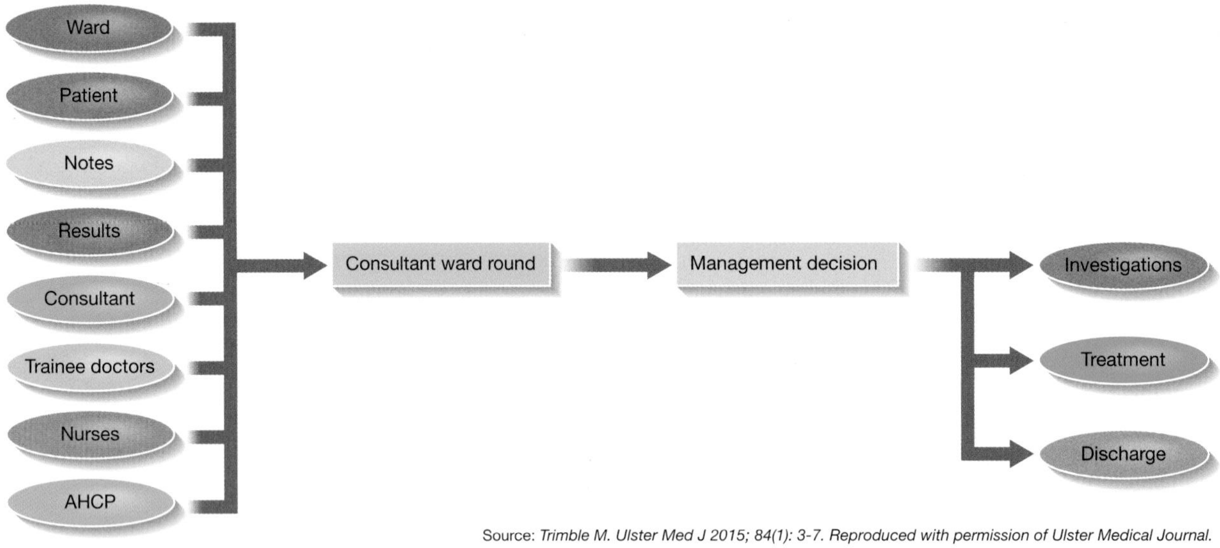

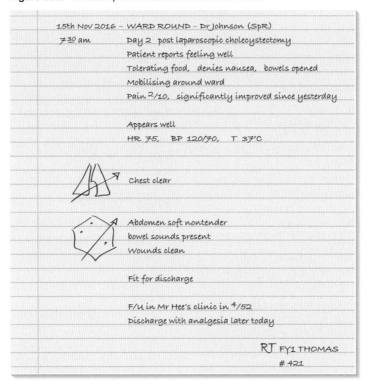

```
Ward
Patient
Notes
Results                    Consultant ward round  →  Management decision      Investigations
Consultant
Trainee doctors                                                               Treatment
Nurses
AHCP                                                                          Discharge
```

Source: *Trimble M. Ulster Med J 2015; 84(1): 3-7. Reproduced with permission of Ulster Medical Journal.*

**Figure 29.2** An example of a documented ward round

> 15th Nov 2016 – WARD ROUND – Dr Johnson (SpR)
>
> 7³⁰ am      Day 2 post laparoscopic cholecystectomy
>
> Patient reports feeling well
>
> Tolerating food, denies nausea, bowels opened
>
> Mobilising around ward
>
> Pain 2/10, significantly improved since yesterday
>
> Appears well
>
> HR 75, BP 120/70, T 37°C
>
> Chest clear
>
> Abdomen soft nontender
>
> bowel sounds present
>
> Wounds clean
>
> Fit for discharge
>
> F/U in Mr Hee's clinic in 4/52
>
> Discharge with analgesia later today
>
>          RJ FY1 THOMAS
>
>          # 421

## Did you know?

When **documenting**, include:
- **Start of the entry** – date, time, speciality, most senior team member's name and designation
- **End of the entry** – printed name and signature, designation, bleep/contact number

# Recording in patient notes

Patient medical notes are **legal documents.** Remember to treat them as such. The must be **written legibly**, in **ink**, and as **completely** as possible. Remember that these notes can be called on for **evidence in court cases**, and therefore anything you record should be of a suitably **formal standard** for this. Refer to the **GMC for further guidance**, as they have **general principles** on this. Medical schools and local education provider Trusts will have their **own protocols** on record-keeping, so ensure that you become familiar with these too. Learning to **use** and **make medical records** is important. Information recorded should be:

- Factual
- Objective
- Complete
- Clear
- Legible
- Unbiased.

Records should be recorded as **close to the time** that the interaction took place as possible.

Patient notes are the **link** between each team mutually treating the patient to assist with **continuity of care**, and for these reasons it is crucial that the note entries are **clear**, **concise** and **accurate**. Members of the different teams will usually record their clinical interactions in the notes as well, although possibly in different sections or areas.

Different Healthcare Trusts have different systems for how notes should be recorded. There can be a smaller set of notes for the **current inpatient stay**, and a larger set of **historical notes** detailing previous admissions and outpatient appointments. Some notes are scanned to create **electronic versions**. Ensure you become familiar with the **local protocols** for recording patient notes at each of your clinical placements.

When documenting a clinical interaction in the patient notes you should include:

- Your full name
- Your designation – including **medical student**
- Time
- Date
- Signature.

Remember that patient notes are **confidential**, and that patients have a right to **access information** on their own medical care, but this access can be through specific channels within the hospital.

# Documenting procedures

If you try to perform a procedure, such as taking blood, document this, even if you are **unsuccessful**. Do not feel embarrassed about **documenting failed attempts**, as it is important to show that you have tried – particularly as a step in **escalating** to gain more appropriate assistance.

# Documenting ward rounds

It is usually one of the **junior doctors** who document the ward rounds. This is an important part of being a junior doctor, although one that is only minimally covered in some medical schools. As a medical student, **observe** the junior doctors on ward rounds whenever possible, as it will help prepare you for your role as a junior doctor, as well as helping you **learn about conditions** and **management plans**.

The ward round allows each patient to be **individually reviewed,** different aspects of their care **integrated** and then their **progress** noted (Figure 29.1).

There are various frameworks for reviewing and recording patients in ward rounds and as requested on the ward (Figure 29.2). A common *aide-memoire* for recording in the notes is **SOAP**, which structures the documentation as:

- Subjective
- Objective
- Assessment
- Plan.

'Subjective' relates to an **impression** of the patient's condition, in relation to their symptoms and appearance. 'Objective' relates to **clinical measures**, including any investigation results and current vital sign measurements. 'Assessment' relates to the assessed condition or diagnosis, and is often also referred to as the 'impression' or 'clinical impression'. 'Plan' refers to the **management plan** that is proposed for treatment.

Other structures for recording in the notes can be based upon an **ABCDE assessment** of the patient, which is useful when **reviewing** an unwell patient on the ward (see Chapter 18).

**Hints and Tips:**
- Ensure you treat patient all records as **confidential**
- Remember patient records are **legal documents** – treat them as such
- Ensure that the **patient's details** are on **every page** of their notes

# 30 Discharge planning

**Figure 30.1** Hospital medicine is part of a wider health care system, which needs to be carefully considered when the patient is discharged

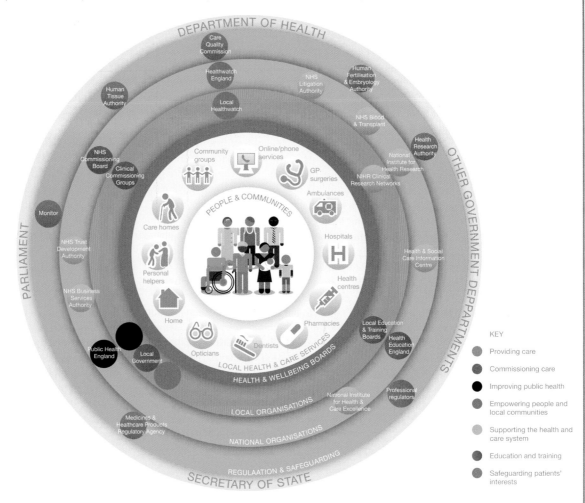

Source: *The health & care system from April 2013.*
*http://webarchive.nationalarchives.gov.uk/20130805112926/http://healthandcare.dh.gov.uk/system-overview-diagram. Used under OGL*

**Hints and Tips:**
- While at medical school, start thinking about what needs to happen to get a patient **safely out of hospital**, aside from management of their immediate health concerns
- Ensure you spend time with **other healthcare professionals**, such as dietitians and pharmacists

# Discharge planning

**Discharge planning** is a very important aspect of a patient's care. It provides the **link** between the patient's hospital admission and their move back to a home environment (or an intermediate step on the way back to a new home environment). The **aim** for the majority of patients will be to discharge them home. This involves all the **steps required** to safely have a patient move from the ward back into their home environment, and should start being considered **well prior** to the day of discharge (Figure 30.1). Begin to think about these aspects when at medical school, as this can help you with understanding about the **continuity of care** that is required.

For example, if an elderly patient is being discharged home, they may need transport to be booked, a home assessment from the occupational therapist or dosset boxes for medication. All of these requirements have various **component steps** – such as request forms – which need to be completed, with **different time frames** and delays. As a student, you may be able to help suggest aspects of the **timing** for this planning and be involved in discussions with other teams (such as the physiotherapists) about this.

Patients are usually provided with **discharge summaries**, which are letters explaining their **diagnosis** and the **treatment** they received. One copy of the discharge summary is usually **sent directly** to their usual **healthcare practitioner** or **GP**. The patient may also receive medications to **take home**, commonly called TTOs, or TTAs ('to take out', or 'to take away', respectively).

As a **junior doctor**, you will be **directly involved** in the discharge planning for patients. It is an area that is not generally covered extensively in a formal way at medical school, but nevertheless comprises a large part of a junior doctor's daily job. Therefore, becoming aware of discharge planning as early as you can in your studies can be of benefit. **Protocols** vary in different hospitals, but discharge summaries and TTOs are usually prepared on a computer – therefore sometimes parts can be completed in advance of an upcoming discharge. As a medical student, you may be able to carry around printed copies of the summaries during ward rounds to help the doctors as they **check** that they are current, and this can help guide your learning on conditions and treatments.

## Explaining discharge summaries

Discharge summaries are **explained fully** to the patient before they go home. They must be **clinically correct**, and **communicated sensitively** to the patient. Discharge summaries are often also used for **coding conditions** for the hospital's records to help **determine costs** for the hospital. This means that **co-morbidities** such as obesity are included on the summary. Ensure that all aspects of a discharge summary are communicated carefully to the patient – not doing so can cause concern in a patient. For instance, if a patient is unaware that they are obese, and they read this on the co-morbidity summary without it having been previously explained to them, they can rightly be surprised and perhaps distressed.

Observing the explanation of discharge summaries to a patient is a good way to develop your **communication skills**, as well as to learn clinical theory– you may even be able to help explain some summaries **under supervision** if permitted by your medical school protocols. Always ensure that a senior doctor **closely** supervises you and also **fully explains** the summary to the patient to ensure the patient is **fully informed.**

Remember that as a medical student you are **not authorised** to discharge a patient from hospital.

If **investigation results** are included in the summary, consultants may prefer the important aspects of the results to be summarised rather than simply pasting the entire report. This then enables any **important findings** to be highlighted for the patient, as well as for any healthcare professionals involved in future care.

At discharge, it is also important to ensure that the patient understands their **medications**, when to seek emergency help and what the **expected follow-up** with their GP or other practitioners will be, if this is required. Observing other doctors conveying this information, and doing it yourself when permitted and supervised, can greatly assist your overall learning and communication skills.

## Medications on TTOs

**Learning doses** and **medication names** from discharge summaries, after having seen the patient during their admission, can be of great assistance to you. Be sure to check doses and interactions in the BNF, and if you are concerned that there are **errors** in the prescribing, discuss it with the appropriate colleague. Even as a student, you have a **duty** to speak up if you think there are any errors or omissions in the medications.

**Controlled medications**, such as morphine, require a different type of prescription to the commonly used electronic prescription. These depend on local protocols, but can require being **countersigned** by hand by the prescribing doctor.

Basic considerations, such as the **opening hours** of the hospital pharmacy, can impact on how long a patient has to wait for discharge. Some teams prepare prescriptions in advance, for regular medications, where this is safe and possible. Medications that are no longer required by the patient are usually stopped or highlighted to the patient's usual GP or healthcare practitioner, if appropriate. As a student you are not authorised to stop these, but do **call attention** to anything you think should have been stopped but has not been.

Also, start thinking about the **interactions** of various medications, and the impact of **poly-pharmacy**, while you are a student (see Chapter 28).

# 31 Managing the acutely unwell patient

**Figure 31.1** The ABCDE approach

| Underlying principles |
|---|
| The approach to all deteriorating or critically ill patients is the same. The underlying principles are: |
| 1. Use the **A**irway, **B**reathing, **C**irculation, **D**isability, **E**xposure (ABCDE) approach to assess and treat the patient |
| 2. Do a complete initial assessment and re-assess regularly |
| 3. Treat life-threatening problems before moving to the next part of assessment |
| 4. Assess the effects of treatment |
| 5. Recognise when you will need extra help. Call for appropriate help early |
| 6. Use all members of the team. This enables interventions (e.g. assessment, attaching monitors, intravenous access), to be undertaken simultaneously |
| 7. Communicate effectively – use the **S**ituation, **B**ackground, **A**ssessment, **R**ecommendation (SBAR) or **R**eason, **S**tory, **V**ital signs, **P**lan (RSVP) approach |
| 8. The aim of the initial treatment is to keep the patient alive, and achieve some clinical improvement. This will buy time for further treatment and making a diagnosis |
| 9. Remember – it can take a few minutes for treatments to work, so wait a short while before reassessing the patient after an intervention |

Source: *Reproduced with permission of Technology Enhanced Learning, University of Portsmouth.*

**Figure 31.2** ALERT™ algorithm for managing the acutely unwell patient

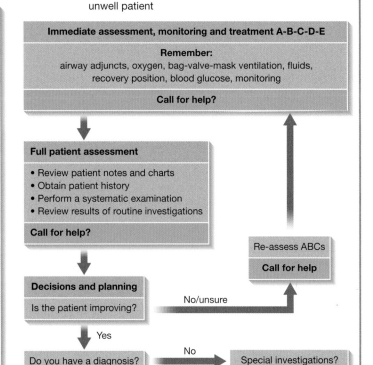

Source: *Professor Gary Smith and colleagues at Portsmouth Hospitals NHS Trust, ALERT™ (http://www.alert-course.com).*

## Managing the acutely unwell patient on the ward

Begin learning about how to manage an **acutely unwell patient** as soon as possible at medical school. **Shadowing** the Senior House Officer or Foundation Year 1 (SHO or FY1) **on-call** and on the **wards** will help you to understand what needs to be done when managing the unwell patient, as will reading **local** and **national protocols**.

When approaching any patient, ask yourself 'Do I need help?' **As a medical student, and even at foundation doctor level, the answer is 'yes'. Ask for help early**, and **call immediately** for an SHO, Specialist Registrar (SpR) or Consultant.

## Getting help on the ward

Frequently, as a **junior doctor** and possibly as a medical student, you might be asked to help call the senior doctor for assistance.

**Handover** is when you give a brief description of what is going on with the patient. There are various approaches, a popular one being the **SBAR** approach.

**S is for Situation** This is a brief summary of what has happened so far (e.g. 'I was called to assess Mr Kay of Willow Ward who has worsening shortness of breath').

**B is for Background** This is a summary of the relevant medical history (e.g. 'Mr Kay is 42 and has a background of COPD. He was admitted 2 days ago with a presumed infective exacerbation').

*Medical School at a Glance*, First Edition. Rachel K. Thomas © 2017 John Wiley & Sons, Ltd. Published 2017 by John Wiley & Sons, Ltd.

**A is for Assessment** This is what you have seen on examination, or what you have been informed of (e.g. 'On assessment he is tachypnoeic, has $SaO_2$ of 88% on air and poor air entry at both lung bases. He does not have a temperature or calf tenderness. His most recent ECG shows sinus tachycardia with no evidence of ST changes. CXR yesterday showed left lower zone pneumonia. The ABG shows a pH of 7.21, $PCO_2$ of 10.1').

**R is for Recommendation** This is what you would like to happen (e.g. 'The SHO asked me to call and would like you to come and help assess this patient as he thinks he has a worsening of his LRTI and might need a repeat CXR and non-invasive ventilation').

As a medical student it is **unlikely** that you will need to do this. However, if you were asked to call on a senior for an unwell patient:

• Be **polite** over the phone. The bleep is the bane of many a doctor's existence! When you call, the doctor might sound busy.

• Say **where** you are calling from (e.g. Willow Ward) and **on behalf** of whom (e.g. the FY1/SHO/Consultant).

• Ask if it is **all right** to speak to them (the senior doctor might be performing a procedure or be with another sick patient, so might not have the capacity to listen or take down the patient's details).

• You might not have all the details about the patient but say briefly why you are calling them. This can be as simple as 'I was asked to call you by Tom the FY1 who is tending to Mr Kay whose shortness of breath is getting worse. He is attending to him at the moment and asked me to call you as he needs some help.'

• Ensure you have **understood** what they would like you to do, and what they are going to do. Are they coming? Do they want you to call someone else?

• **Feedback** to the person who asked you to make the call that you have made it and what the outcome was.

## Managing an unwell patient

**Management** is delivered in a structured **ABCDE approach** (as is the **assessment**) (see Chapter 18). **Always ask for help early. Examination and emergency management are usually carried out together**, although they have been partially separated in these chapters to facilitate learning. **Always adhere to current local and national protocols and guidelines, which are updated frequently, and resources such as www.Resus.org.uk** (Figures 31.1 and 31.2). The framework described here is to help you to start structuring your learning and thinking. This is a sample of how you could think about management, and is not intended as a comprehensive guide.

**A is for Airway** Clear the airway, if it is obstructed, with **manoeuvres** (e.g. jaw thrust, chin lift and head tilt), **suction**, or **insertion** of a naso- or oro-pharyngeal airway). Does the patient need **oxygen**? Give oxygen to maintain saturations of 94–98% (or of 88–92% if the patient is at risk of hypercapnic failure).

**B is for Breathing** Is there any difficulty in breathing? Examine the chest to try to find a treatable source (e.g. chronic obstructive pulmonary disorder, asthma, congestive cardiac failure or pulmonary embolism). If you identify a treatable source and it is **life threatening, treat it immediately**. Is breathing within the normal rate of 12–20 breaths/min, and is chest expansion symmetrical? A **high respiratory rate (RR)** signifies **severe illness** and a **risk of deterioration**. Support with bag-valve-mask ventilation, or non-invasive ventilation if required.

**C is for Circulation** Examine the heart. What is their **heart rate** and the **rhythm**? Do you need to formally assess the rhythm (e.g. ECG)? What is their blood pressure and capillary refill time? Are there signs of bleeding or sepsis that can be treated?

Do you need a fluid bolus? Are they hypovolaemic? Are they passing urine? **Insert large-bore cannulae** for high flow delivery of fluids. Take blood samples and give fluids if indicated according to local and national protocols, and the clinical picture. **Immediately treat life-threatening conditions**, such as acute coronary syndrome (ACS).

**D is for Disability** If their Glasgow Coma Score (GCS)/AVPU is reduced, what is the cause? Look at their pupils, and on the drug chart (e.g. are opioids involved?) Measure their blood **glucose level**, and treat any **hypoglycaemia** according to **local** and **national protocols** if it is present (e.g. below 4.0 mmol/L). If the patient is **unconscious** and their airway is not protected, place them in the **lateral position.**

**E is for Exposure** While respecting the patient's dignity, expose and examine them as required.

**Start initial management.** This can be as simple as giving some oxygen or asking for a bedside investigation.

Consider what **investigations** you might need:

• *Bedside tests:* urinalysis, ECG

• *Blood tests:* full blood count (FBC), urea and electrolytes (U&Es), liver function test (LFT), C-reactive protein (CRP), group and save (G&S), venous blood gas (VBG), arterial blood gas (ABG)

• *Radiology:* chest X-ray, CT head, CT pulmonary angiogram, abdominal X-ray.

## Admitting a patient to ITU

The management of an acutely unwell patient can usually be carried out on the ward, but occasionally the patient needs to be taken to an **intensive care/therapy unit (ICU/ITU)** or a **high dependency unit (HDU)**. Every ITU is different and will have **different thresholds** for admitting patients depending on the facilities available in the hospital. If you think that your patient will need more support or is at risk of deteriorating, think about letting the ITU team **know in advance** so that they can come to review them. Often, they will review and suggest ways of **optimising** the patient's care on the ward.

Admitting a patient to ITU means a **liaison** between the team looking after the patient, often involving the consultant in charge of the patient (medical or surgical), the intensive care team, nurses, and the patient or representative of the patient (e.g. relative or named family member). Usually, this is a discussion on the reasons for admission, the management of foreseeable events and what the patient would like to happen. As a medical student, this is a useful discussion to observe so that you can learn first-hand about the management of sick patients.

Reasons to admit patients to ITU:

• For high level nursing care

• For invasive monitoring that cannot be carried out on the ward

• Being identified at risk of deteriorating

• After a high-risk procedure

• For a definitive airway

• For invasive breathing assistance

• Reduced/falling/variable GCS

• For haemodialysis or haemofiltration.

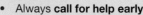

**Hints and Tips:**

• Always **call for help early**
• Remember that the larger the gauge number of a cannula, the smaller the diameter of its lumen

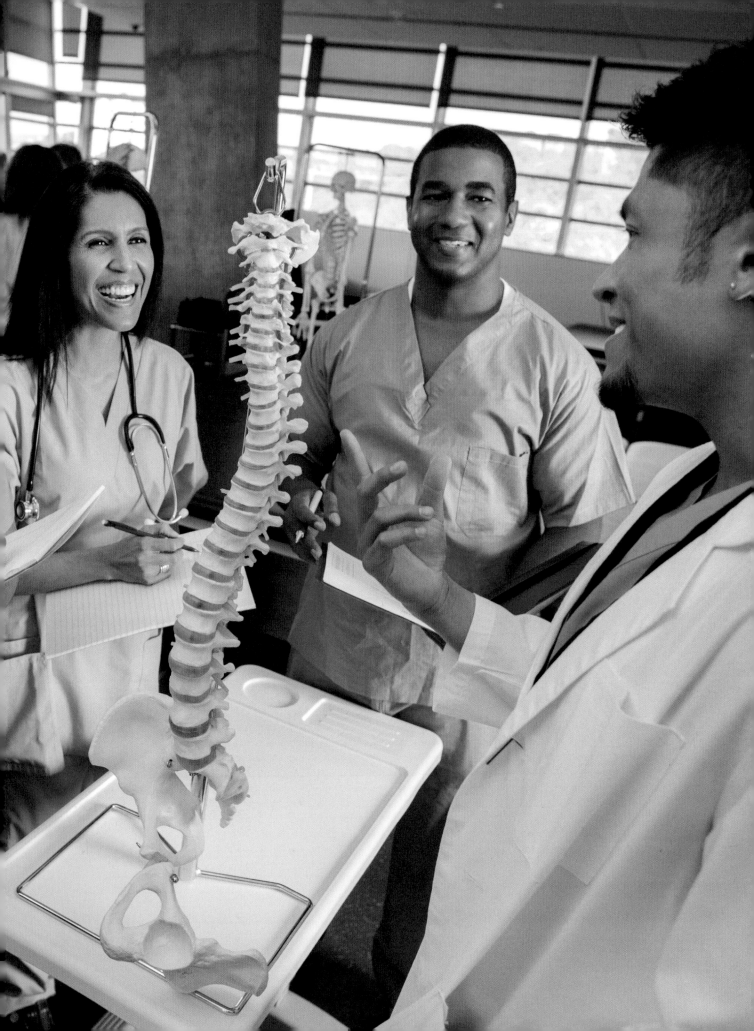

# Completing medical school

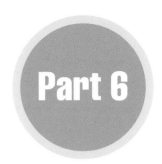

**Part 6**

## Chapters

# 32 Examinations

**Figure 32.1** An example of an on-line question – ensure that you read all questions carefully, and note the marking schemes!

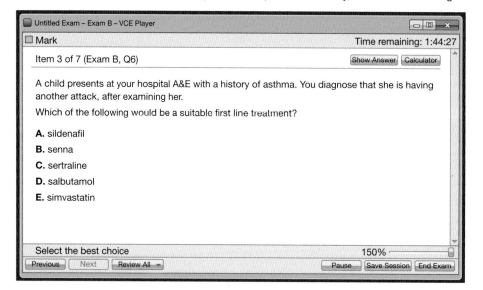

**Figure 32.2** Clinical examinations

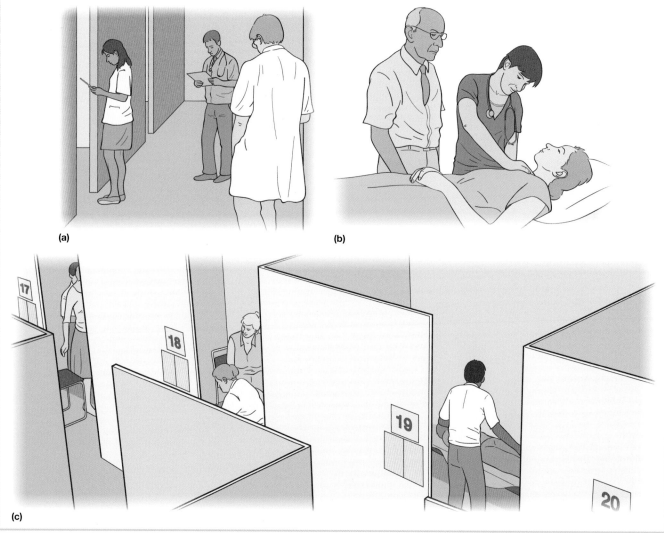

## Written examinations

The structure and frequency of examinations at medical school vary depending on which university you attend and the year you are in. Generally, the examinations include both written and clinical components.

Written examinations vary in format: essay questions, short answer questions or single word answers.

Ensure that you note the **marking scheme** for each question, and divide your time accordingly.

## Online examinations

Many medical schools have examination components that are **online** (Figure 32.1). The examinations are often multiple-choice questions (MCQs), single best answers (SBQs) or extended matching questions (EMQs). This online format offers several advantages. It enables high-resolution images to be viewed (at a fraction of the environmental and financial cost of traditional paper printing), and quick, efficient marking.

As with any examination, prepare by working through **previous exams.** Ensure that you are familiar with the layout of the questions and how to use the equipment. Be careful, as at times scrolling down the 'page' using the mouse scroll-button can change previously selected answers. If possible, use the arrow buttons on the keyboard instead. Also take care to ensure that, where you initially do not answer a question, you return to it later. Prior to the exam find out whether there will be negative marking for wrong answers.

Many online examinations have a countdown or clock somewhere visible on the screen so, as with any exam, ensure that you pay attention to time management and do not dwell for a disproportionately long time on any one question (unless the marks indicate that you should).

Many online examinations are held in **computer labs.** If they are taken at home, ensure that you have an adequate internet connection, a suitably up-to-date browser and enough time to sit and concentrate.

## Open-book examinations

A few examinations in medical school are **open book**. If you have this type of exam, do not be lulled into thinking that it requires no study. They can be difficult, as time can be spent leafing through pages of texts, inevitably becoming distracted as you find something interesting to read (that you should have studied already!). Additional preparation for open-book assessments involves marking key areas of the text for quick access.

## Viva voce

If you do not pass an exam, or your answers are concerning to the marker, you may be offered a **viva voce** (viva). These vivas are really just a chance to show how much you do actually know. Their structure depends on different medical schools, but usually consist of answering questions from a panel of academics or lecturers. In order to prepare for these, continue studying and perhaps speak with tutors or students who were given vivas if your medical school allows this. Occasionally, vivas will also be held for exceptional students, in order to decide who will be awarded a **prize**. It

goes without saying that you should have an idea of which candidate you are – and if you do not, ask!

## Clinical examinations

Most medical schools use **objective structured clinical examinations** (OSCEs) to examine clinical skills. These are usually divided up into medical and surgical OSCEs. Each of these is divided up into stations (Figure 32.2). Each station has a specific **marking scheme** for the examiner to follow, in an effort to minimise subjective elements in these exams.

Most medical schools make their marking scheme available to students, so make yourself aware of what is required. There are usually components such as **failure to wash your hands,** which result in an immediate fail for a station – no matter how well you perform in other areas.

After the clinical examination of the required system, you will often be asked to present the findings (see Chapter 25), a differential diagnosis (see Chapter 24), investigations (see Chapter 23) and a management plan. When you are put on the spot, it can be difficult to remember aspects such as causes for a disease – remember to use tools such as your **surgical sieve** (see Chapter 24). There can also be stations on communication (see Chapter 9) or breaking bad news (see Chapter 27).

Ensure that you wear the appropriate **clinical dress**, as you would for any patient interaction (see Chapter 3). Ensure you check the medical school's guidelines for the correct clothing for clinical examinations well in advance.

## General advice

It is normal to feel **stressed** around exam time – particularly if the exam counts significantly towards you passing the course. Some medical schools weigh in-course assessments more heavily than others but, irrespective of this, the end-of-placement written papers and clinical examinations still usually need to be **passed**.

At exam time it can be tempting to feel that you must spend every spare hour studying, but remember to make time to **eat, sleep** and **relax**. Exercise is a great stress release. **Taking time out** for other activities will mean you are more effective when you sit at your desk.

While passing examinations seems a major focus at medical school, there is a reason that there is only one chapter devoted to them in this book. Exams are really just a **checkpoint** to ensure that you are on the right track with your learning. Regarding them in this way helps diffuse the pressure that can sometimes be associated with them. Examinations are a part of life as a doctor, but they are just a part, not the focus. Try to keep them in **perspective** when they are looming near, and seek additional support if you feel that you need it (see Chapter 5).

**Hints and Tips:**
- Try to enjoy some **leisure time** while sitting exams
- **Read all examination questions carefully**
- Ensure that you **allocate** your time during examinations properly

# 33 Electives and special study modules

**Figure 33.1** Medical electives enable exposure to a broad range of other medical systems

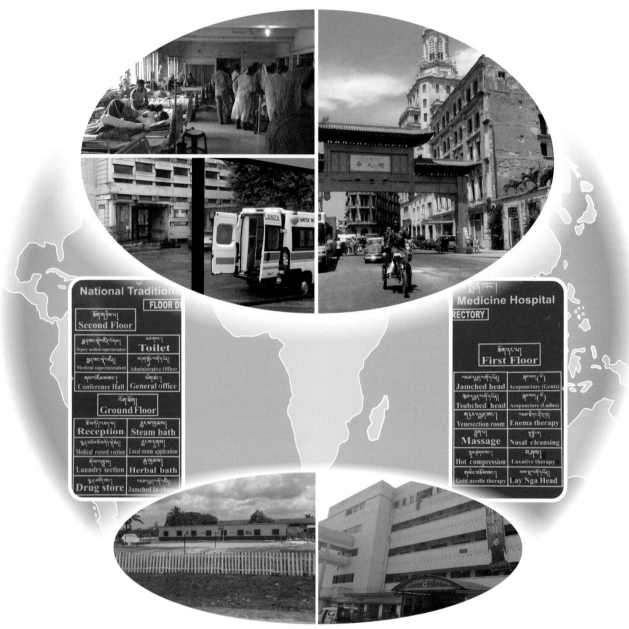

Source: *Images courtesy of: Dr Rachel Thomas (images of hospital in Italy and Cuba). Dr Alexander Kumar (image of floor plan of hospital in Bhutan), and Nicholas May (images of ward and exterior of hospital in Bangladesh).*

**Did you know?**

It is important to ensure that you **debrief** and **reflect** after you return home from your ME, irrespective of whether you spent it in a low, middle or high-income country.
This can help:
- Support you with any **cultural, ethical** or **clinical** issues that you have encountered
- Help guide your **learning**
- **Improve** your future clinical practice
- Help **minimise similar issues** for future students

# Electives

A highly anticipated period of time occurs towards the end of medical school with the **medical elective** (ME), which lasts usually **6–12 weeks**. For your ME, you arrange a placement at a **host institution** other than where you are undertaking your degree. Many students choose to take their electives **abroad**, often in low or middle income countries (Figure 33.1).

MEs **vary** greatly between medical schools, in relation to **timing**, **length** and **assessment requirements**. Some medical schools have MEs that are **pass/fail** components of the course, while others require a **poster**, a **presentation** or an **essay** to be submitted at the end. Most MEs have the requirement for a supervisor to **sign off** that you have **completed it satisfactorily**.

People select MEs for different reasons. Some students choose areas of their **career interest**, while others choose exotic locations for a sense of **adventure**. The ME can also be an opportunity to learn more about other areas of medicine that are less fully covered at medical school, such as **Global Health**.

Defining your **objectives** prior to starting your ME can help you maximise the value that you gain from your elective. You then have some direction for deciding on where would be a **suitable location**, and guidance on relevant activities for the ME. Finding a **suitable ME supervisor** is also important.

When travelling to areas outside the UK, do not forget to consider matters such as **risk, safety** and **ethics**. Your medical school will usually have thorough **pre-departure training** on these points. Another important point to consider is the **impact** you may have on the host institution. It is common to assume that this will only be positive, but there are **negative impacts** associated with hosting elective students. Your presence can **drain resources** or disturb **fragile healthcare infrastructures**.

It is also important to ensure that you do not practise outside your **competencies**, and that you have support available to deal with any problems or **ethical dilemmas** that may arise. **Pre-departure**, it is a good idea to spend time considering and discussing potential issues, and to devise a framework for dealing with them if they do arise. For **safety**, as well as for **learning** and **reflection** purposes, you may wish to undertake your ME with another student.

**Reflection** improves learning, so consider including this even if it is not stipulated as a requirement of your assessment. **Reciprocity** is also an important element for you to consider, even if it is not formally included in your ME by your medical school. Think about how you could give back to your host institution. Some students do this by taking equipment and books, or assisting with tutorials at their host placement.

**Funding** can often be a barrier for MEs abroad. However, there are avenues to help with funding – for example, medical schools may have scholarships, and various charities provide bursaries.

It can be helpful to ask **previous students** in the years above you about their ME experiences. Research the **resources** that your medical school has available. It is a good idea to prepare yourself with as much knowledge on **local practices**, **culture**, **language** and **expectations** of the location you are travelling to for your ME, before you embark on what should be an enriching experience.

# Special study modules

**Special study modules** (SSMs) are areas of study that you select with the syllabus. They usually run for shorter periods of time such as **2–4 weeks** and offer you the opportunity to learn more about a **specific area** of medicine.

Generally, these modules can be **self-arranged** or selected from a **more formal** set of arrangements already organised by your medical school. The format **varies** with different medical schools. If you are interested in a particular area for which your medical school has no SSM, they may be open to your arranging your own, if you can persuade them that it would be beneficial for your future career.

SSMs, which are sometimes referred to as **student-selected components** or **student-selected modules**, include placements in fields such as anaesthetics, addiction psychiatry and medical publishing.

As with MEs, the **timing**, **duration** and **assessment** requirements of SSMs vary among medical schools. Ensure that you know what is expected of you, as SSMs can be an essential part of the **curriculum** that must be **passed**.

# General advice

As with most areas of medicine – and indeed life – **being organised** streamlines the **planning** and **execution** of MEs and SSMs. Be **enthusiastic** when contacting potential supervisors. Find out as much information as you can, so that you can form realistic **expectations** and set appropriate **objectives**.

After your initial periods of interaction with the doctors and other students while you are on MEs and SSMs, try to maintain these **professional relationships** after the module concludes. Ensure that you thank people appropriately. You may be surprised at the assistance you can offer each other during your future careers.

**Hints and Tips:**
- Consider your **impact** on your host institution
- Try to include aspects such as **reciprocity** and **reflection**
- **Discuss** with previous students
- **Define** your **objectives**
- **Continue relationships** built in both medical electives and special study modules

# 34 Understanding foundation school

**Figure 34.1** Aim of the Foundation Programme

The Foundation Programme is a 2-year structured, supervised programme of workplace-based learning for medical school graduates, which exists to prepare junior doctors for specialty training by providing them with the medical knowledge and skills to meet the requirements of the GMC's *The New Doctor and the Foundation Programme Curriculum*. The programme is designed to provide foundation doctors with the ability to reflect on their aspirations and attributes and match these with service need.

Source: *www.foundationprogramme.nhs.uk*

**Table 34.1 (a)** Educational performance measure (EPM) marks break-down
**(b)** Situational judgement test (SJT) marks break-down

The EPM is worth a maximum of 50 points and is comprised of three parts:

| EPM component | Number of points |
|---|---|
| Medical school performance (calculated in deciles) | 34–43 |
| Additional degrees | 0–5 |
| Other educational achievements | 0–2 |
| Maximum number of points available | 50 |

**(a)**

Distribution of SJT scores for Foundation Programme 2015

| SJT points | Applicants (%) |
|---|---|
| 0.00–10.00 | 0.04 |
| 10.01–20.00 | 0.20 |
| 20.01–30.00 | 2.82 |
| 30.01–35.00 | 13.18 |
| 35.01–40.00 | 45.20 |
| 40.01–45.00 | 36.47 |
| 45.01–50.00 | 2.09 |

**(b)** Source: *www.foundationprogramme.nhs.uk*

**Table 34.2** Supervised learning events (SLEs) and assessments are required for each placement

Recommended minimum number of SLEs per placement

| Supervised learning event | Recommended minimum number per placement* |
|---|---|
| Direct observation of doctor/ patient interaction: | |
| Mini-CEX | 3 or more |
| DOPS | Optional to supplement mini-CEX |
| Case-based discussion (CBD) | 2 or more |
| Developing the clinical teacher | 1 or more |

Frequency of assessments

| Assessments | Frequency |
|---|---|
| E-portfolio | Contemporaneous |
| Core procedures | Throughout F1 |
| Team assessment of behaviour (TAB) | Once in first placement in both F1 and F2, optional repitition |
| Clinical supervisor's end of placement report | Once per placement |
| Educational supervisor's end of placement report | Once per placement |
| Educational supervisor's end of end of year report | Once per year |

* Based on a clinical placement of 4 months' duration

Source *www.foundationprogramme.nhs.uk*

**Figure 34.2** Possible aspects of reflective practice

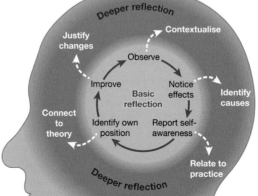

*Medical School at a Glance*, First Edition. Rachel K. Thomas © 2017 John Wiley & Sons, Ltd. Published 2017 by John Wiley & Sons, Ltd.

After medical school, the next phase of training is in the **Foundation Programme,** which is co-ordinated by the **UK Foundation Programme Office** (UKFPO) (Figure 34.1). This **2-year programme** is compulsory, with formal assessments of progress at the end of each year. **Full GMC registration** is achieved after satisfactory completion of Foundation Year 1 (FY1), and a successful **Annual Review of Competence Progression** (ARCP).

## Foundation Programme application

In the final year of medical school, the **online applications** for the Foundation Programme open on the **Foundation Programme Application System** (FPAS). The application process is **competitive.** The application can be made for one of the **two streams** – the Foundation Programme or the Academic Foundation Programme.

The application consists of several parts, including the **Educational Performance Measure** (EPM), and the **Situational Judgement Test** (SJT). The EPM tests for skills (both clinical and non-clinical) and knowledge. The SJT tests for desirable attributes and judgement.

The Academic Foundation Programme usually also includes an **interview,** with this being decided by their own criteria.

As part of the application process, you rank your preference of Foundation School. There are 26 to rank, with the highest scoring applicants allocated their first choice – moving down through subsequent choices as the positions in each Foundation School fill.

The application is scored out of 100 (Table 34.1). This mark is a combination of how you perform on the assessment and in the application process, and on a ranking within your medical school.

The aims of the Foundation Programme include:
- Building on medical school education
- Providing generic training
- Developing leadership
- Providing various experiences to help inform career choices.

## Foundation learning portfolios

Your progress through each year is recorded online, in the **Foundation learning electronic portfolio** (e-portfolio). This enables aspects such as the **supervised learning events** (SLEs) to be captured (Table 34.2). Your e-portfolio forms the basis for your **appraisal** at the end of each year, and you can also use it in the future for supporting your applications for future training and employment.

You must also keep a **paper portfolio.** This consists of a printout of the e-portfolio, along with any certificates and evidence of other learning. Start adding to this as soon as you can, and keep it up to date. It is much easier to remove any unnecessary items later rather than to try to find all your documentation when your assessment is due.

## Foundation Programme curriculum

Satisfactory completion of the Foundation Programme is linked to an **outcome-based curriculum**.

It has key messages, including:
- Patient safety
- Personal development.

Specific aspects should be met, such as:
- Supervised learning events
- Competence in core procedures
- 360° team assessment of behaviour feedback.

Aspects such as **reflective practice** (Figure 34.2) and **quality improvement projects** are highly regarded.

## Foundation Year 1

Foundation Year 1 focuses on increasing and improving the knowledge and skills you have gained at medical school. It enables you to take **supervised responsibility** in the management of patients.

## Foundation Year 2

Foundation Year 2 (FY2) focuses on building on the knowledge and skills gained in FY1, giving you **increasing responsibility** for the care of patients. At the satisfactory completion of FY2, you are awarded a **Foundation Achievement of Competence Document** (FACD). This document shows that you are ready to begin a training programme for specialty, core or general practice.

## Supervised learning events

Supervised learning events (SLEs) with the patient include:
- Mini-clinical evaluation exercise (mini-CEX)
- Direct observation of procedural skills (DOPs).

Supervised learning events (SLEs) without the patient include:
- Case-based discussion (CBD)
- Developing the clinical teacher.

You are required to complete a **minimum number** of SLEs in order to gain sign-off, with the specific number set each year. Generally, the requirements are for more than nine directly observed encounters (mini-CEX and DOPS, with more than six mini-CEX), more than six CBDs, and one Developing the clinical teacher.

## Assessment

Your assessment, and **subsequent sign-off**, is based on:
- Your competency in core procedures
- Evidence shown in your e-portfolio of SLEs and other activities
- Team assessment of your behaviour (TAB)
- End of placement reports from your Clinical Supervisor, and end of placement and end of year reports from your Educational Supervisor (see Chapter 3).

The TAB is an online assessment of your behaviour, from approximately 10 members of the multi-disciplinary team, such as consultants, nurses and occupational therapists. Usually, a minimum of one of these must be completed in each year.

**Hints and Tips:**
- **Familiarise** yourself with the curriculum and start working through it **early**
- Add as much as you can to your paper portfolio – you can always take it out later
- Keep your portfolio **up to date**, to save you rushing to fill it at the end of the year

# 35 Understanding later training

**Figure 35.1** Steps in a clinical medical career

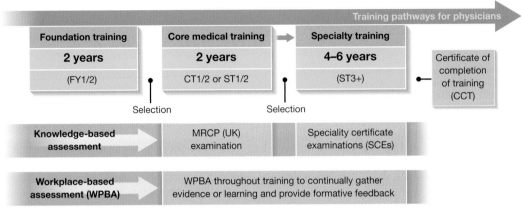

Source: Based on https://www.rcpe.ac.uk/careers-training/specialty-training-guide

**Figure 35.2** Steps in a clinical academic career

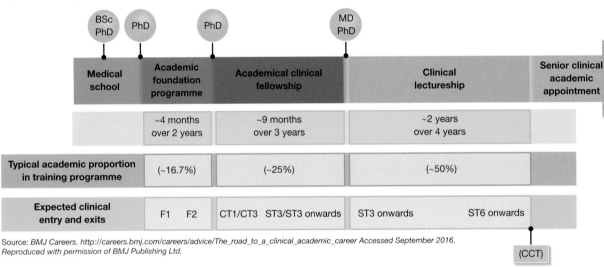

Source: BMJ Careers. http://careers.bmj.com/careers/advice/The_road_to_a_clinical_academic_career Accessed September 2016. Reproduced with permission of BMJ Publishing Ltd.

**Hints and Tips:**
- **Decline positions** as soon as you know you will not be accepting them
- Use **taster weeks** in your training to explore specialties that you may be interested in
- Check **Specialty Training websites** for current information on application processes

**Figure 35.3** Options to take time out of traditional training

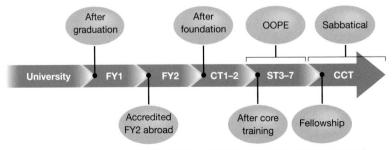

Source: Based on http://www.theadventuremedic.com/features/taking-time-out-from-uk-training/

*Medical School at a Glance*, First Edition. Rachel K. Thomas © 2017 John Wiley & Sons, Ltd. Published 2017 by John Wiley & Sons, Ltd.

During FY2, you are able to apply for **specialty** and **core training** (see Chapter 3). Depending on the training that you complete, this later enables you to **practise independently** as a Consultant or a GP. At the end of the training, you are awarded a **Certificate of Completion of Training** (CCT), and entry to the GMC's specialist or GP **Register** (Figure 35.1).

**Career planning advice** is available from many sources, including Supervisors, Consultants and websites such as Medical Careers (www.medicalcareers.nhs.uk).

You may choose to be involved in research, and apply for an **Academic Clinical Fellowship** (ACF; Figure 35.2). These fellowships, offered within most clinical specialties, combine both clinical and academic duties.

## Specialty and core training application

Applications for specialty (ST) and core training (CT) positions are generally opened in rounds, with Round 1 starting several months into FY2 (Figure 35.1). Any remaining positions are filled by Round 2 occurring several months later. Sites such as Modernising Medical Careers (www.mmc.nhs.uk), NHS jobs (www.jobs.nhs.uk) and **Deanery websites** can be used to help apply for these training positions.

The applications for ACF funding usually close earlier than those for ST or CT roles.

After submission of the **online application form,** you may be shortlisted for an **interview**. If successful in this interview, you will be offered a place on the training programme.

The **time frames** for applications and acceptance of offers of interviews and positions can be quite short, so ensure that you check the requirements carefully. The applications differ between specialties, with the Royal Colleges and Deaneries generally managing the online process.

Specialty training can be **run through** or **uncoupled.**

With run through training, you automatically progress to the next level of training, provided you complete all of the competencies that are required.

Uncoupled training consists of an initial phase of **core training** (CT), usually 2 or 3 years. Once this has been satisfactorily completed, there is competitive application for later training (ST3 or ST4, depending on the number of CT years completed).

It is possible to undertake **less than full time training** (LTFT) during both the Foundation Programme and later training. This can be included on the application form, or discussed with the body responsible for training.

There are also options to **take time out** from later medical training (Figure 35.3). These options should be discussed directly with the Deanery or Royal College.

## Portfolios

Portfolios are required to **support** any applications, and are frequently viewed at the interview. It is important to keep them **up-to-date**. Include anything in your portfolio that might help distinguish you from other applicants. Evidence of **continued learning**, such as certificates from online modules or courses that you have attended, as well as **thank you letters** or **cards from patients,** can be included.

**Reflective practice** – reflecting on what went well, and what did not go as well as you had hoped – should be a key part of all practice. It can help **improve future practice,** as well as helping you chart your **progress.** You should also include evidence of reflective practice in your portfolio.

Your portfolio can be used to show a continued interest in, or **commitment** to, a specialty or area of particular interest. This can be reinforced by including evidence of presentations, teaching, papers or attendance at Grand Rounds in the relevant area.

## Interviews

Ensure that you **prepare well** for your interview. This includes gaining permission for **time off work,** planning how to travel to the interview and gathering the supporting evidence for your application. Ensure that you are clear about where the interview will be held, and that you have thought through answers to possible interview questions. While all this sounds like common sense, it can be easy to forget when under pressure!

Common question themes include:
- Why are you interested in this area?
- Why should we choose you?
- Why is teaching/clinical governance/audit important?
- What would you do in this clinical situation?

## Assessments

You are also required to complete the **Annual Review of Competence Progression** (ARCP) during the training programmes. An up-to-date portfolio is key in completing ARCPs.

During these later phases of training you are required to take your **membership examinations.** These examinations are **expensive** and **time-consuming,** and have a **low pass rate.** The timing and structure of the examinations vary depending on the area of study. The application process also varies within each area. Generally, the examinations take several months of intense preparation, and must be applied for several months in advance. They are generally divided into two or three sections, covering both written and practical assessments.

For example, medicine's **Membership of the Royal College of Physicians** (MRCP) involves:
- Part 1 written science examination
- Part 2 written clinical paper
- PACES clinical examination.

Surgery's **Membership of the Royal College of Surgeons** (MRCS) has:
- Part A written science examination
- Part B clinical examination.

# 36 Other uses for medical degrees

**Figure 36.1** There are a variety of careers, apart from clinical medicine, where a medical degree is helpful

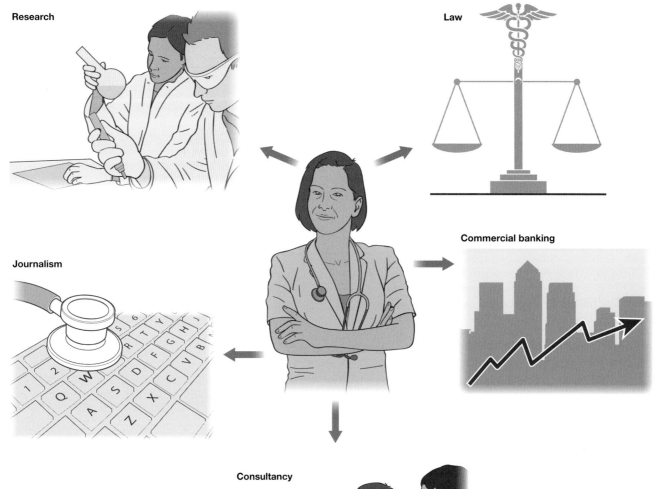

Research

Law

Commercial banking

Journalism

Consultancy

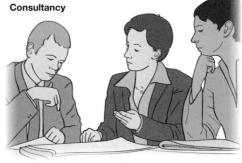

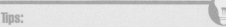

**Hints and Tips:**
- Ask for **careers advice early**
- Investigate the broad range of career options available within the **clinical setting**
- Investigate options within the **academic setting**
- Investigate other options in the **wider fields** of other occupations – a **medical degree** will stand you in good stead **for many careers**

*Medical School at a Glance*, First Edition. Rachel K. Thomas © 2017 John Wiley & Sons, Ltd. Published 2017 by John Wiley & Sons, Ltd.

# Other uses for a medical degree

The field of medicine encompasses a **wide variety** of careers. Although you may be tempted to think doctors fall into one of only a few categories of specialties or roles, such as hospital doctor or GP, the range of potential positions is wider than you may imagine (Figure 36.1). Some people realise that clinical medicine is not for them, or prefer a change and pursue a career in another area. It is encouraging to know that by completing a medical degree, you are in a **strong position** to be successful in many careers.

You may consider having a degree largely unrelated to the position for which you are applying as something that will work against you but this is not necessarily the case. Possessing a medical degree and working for even a short period in the medical field demonstrates **key skills. Academic prowess**, **team-working skills** and **problem-solving ability** are all requisites for becoming a doctor and many employers will infer you have these attributes from your medical degree alone. This works greatly in your favour, boosting your credentials as a candidate.

So, with the career world your oyster, what avenues are open to you? This is, of course, dependent on your **individual interests** and **personal preferences.** However, there are a number of careers that seem particularly popular with medical graduates.

## Law

A career in **Law** has similarities to a career in medicine in that a **solid academic basis** is required before progression up a hierarchical structure can occur. There is, of course, overlap between the two fields and this is often the inspiration for many doctors to pursue a legal career. **Medicolegal** work encompassing negligence cases, medical defence and the work of the Coroner are roles that benefit from both a doctor's and a lawyer's knowledge. Once you obtain legal qualifications, you then have the foundation to pursue a career in other, non-medical aspects of Law if that is where your interests lie.

## Management consultancy

**Management consultancy** is a system whereby a hired consulting firm **analyses** an organisation's systems, with the purpose of **improving efficiency**, attaining a goal or **problem-solving.** Because of the broad variety of client organisations, the work and projects are diverse. Your problem-solving skills learnt in medical school will be highly valued in this career. In addition, a strong business background such as a Masters in Business Administration is also regarded favourably. As with many 'City jobs', the hours and the rewards with this career can vary considerably.

## Commercial banking

**Commercial banking** has a particular aura and reputation associated with it. A position that involves reviewing organisations' finances and **investing** their assets for maximal profit requires an analytical brain and an ability to make important decisions under **pressure** and uncertainty. As in management consultancy, banking can involve long working hours and a competitive environment. However, the rewards and financial incentives can compensate for this. Your medical degree should suffice in applications for positions but any business or financial experience can boost your application.

## Journalism

**Medical journalism** is a field that can be pursued **concurrently** with a medical career. Being involved in the field you are writing about helps to keep you informed about developments and practices. There are a select number of positions available with noted journals (e.g. the *BMJ*), although these posts are highly coveted. To boost your chances of obtaining such a job, you should start building up evidence in your **writing portfolio.** Writing for smaller papers, or even the hospital you work for in their local bulletins, will start you on your way.

With the rise of blogging, there are increasing opportunities online. Remember that in your position as a doctor there are certain **responsibilities** that apply with the dissemination of information. If you are freelancing, you must make sure that you work within your remit as outlined by the GMC and **maintain confidentiality.**

## Research and pharmaceutical industries

The **research** and **pharmaceutical industries** are aligned with medicine. Many medical degrees actually encompass a research element, so this will help you in applications for positions, particularly if you are able to **publish research papers** from the project.

There are a variety of positions available in these areas and you will need to research them further to find out what appeals to you. Further qualifications and training may be required if you wish to perform **laboratory-based research**, so be prepared for this. Talking to research-orientated professors, while you are still in the medical profession, can guide you as to the next steps in applying for such a job.

## Innovation and entrepreneurship

With the rapid advances in technology, some doctors are moving towards improving current healthcare systems in innovative ways and some are involved in **start-ups.** Debate is taking place on the merits of continuing a career in clinical practice versus focusing solely on medically related technological innovations. The NHS provides a **Clinical Entrepreneur** training programme, which enables training in this rapidly evolving area (https://www.england.nhs.uk/2015/11/11/cent-programme/). There are also other resources available on entrepreneurship, as well as **online support platforms** and **communities.**

## For more information

If you realise that medicine is not for you, or you wish to explore alternative careers, **do your research before applying** for positions. You may wish to discuss your reasons for changing career with a **sympathetic senior,** in case there are small issues that can be addressed that would make you more inclined to stay in medicine.

There are a number of services, such as **alternative career fairs,** which are available for doctors considering a change in direction. A basic **online search** can be a starting point, and a **talk with a career advisor** can also be helpful. Regardless of which career you eventually choose to pursue, remember your medical degree is a **great achievement** and also shows you survived your time as a medical student!

# 37 First day as a doctor

**Figure 37.1** An example of a patient list

| Patient details | Admission details, PMH | Investigation results | | | | | | | | | Jobs |
|---|---|---|---|---|---|---|---|---|---|---|---|
| | | Spinal Team Friday October 17 2016 | | | | | | | | | |
| **Green Ward** | | | | | | | | | | | |
| Dr Brown Side Room 1 | Jenny SMITH #42491 09/02/1982 | 7th Oct: admitted with 10/7 sciatica known L5/S1 prolapse no focal neurology | Date 7/10 8/10 13/10 15/10 | Hb 132 135 133 133 | WCC 3.9 5.1 5.3 5.7 | PLT 194 193 195 196 | Na 138 140 139 139 | K 4.3 4.4 4.3 4.5 | egfr 74 75 74 80 | Cr 75 74 72 69 | VTE forms ✓ ✓ ✓ ✓ | Surgery planned 17th Post op bloods 17th Post op Xray |
| Dr Brown Bed 2 | Sally JONES #73619 08/11/1949 | 15th Oct: admitted for primary excision of cervical intervertebral disc | Date 15/10 16/10 | Hb 135 136 | WCC 5.1 5.1 | PLT 193 194 | Na 140 141 | K 4.4 4.5 | egfr 76 77 | Cr 72 73 | VTE forms ✓ ✓ | Physiotherapy Post op analgesia |
| Dr Brown Bed 5 | Sarah TIMS #82815 12/12/1967 | 15th Oct: admitted for correction of scoliosis | Date 15/10 16/10 | Hb 128 132 | WCC 4.1 4.2 | PLT 160 161 | Na 140 142 | K 4.0 4.1 | egfr 108 110 | Cr 67 69 | VTE forms ✓ ✓ | Post op bloods Post op Xray when mobilising |
| **Yellow Ward** | | | | | | | | | | | |
| Dr Jay Bed 1 | Ben ELLIS #59581 11/11/1972 | 16th Oct: admitted for L4/L5 disc replacement | Date 16/10 | Hb 130 | WCC 4.9 | PLT 163 | Na 140 | K 4.5 | egfr 120 | Cr 75 | VTE forms ✓ | Regular morphine Post op bloods Post op Xray Physiotherapy |
| Dr Jay Bed 5 | Harry CHAPS #72813 13/6/1980 | 14th Oct: progressive numbness & tingling, started in hand → shoulder now severe neck pain | Date 15/10 16/10 | Hb 131 111 | WCC 6.0 7.5 | PLT 168 170 | Na 139 139 | K 4.0 3.8 | egfr 110 115 | Cr 66 67 | VTE forms ✓ ✓ | Continue IV dex. Oncology referral |
| Dr Jay Bed 4 | Simon HIGGS #93814 20/7/1968 | Referral from Dukes. 15th Oct: subdural & epidural abcess On abx | Date 15/10 16/10 | Hb 95 96 | WCC 9.3 10.2 | PLT 580 600 | Na 135 136 | K 4.0 4.2 | egfr 110 109 | Cr 70 70 | VTE forms ✓ ✓ | Microbiology referral Pain team referral Repeat bloods ?PICC line Start pabrinex |

**Figure 37.2** A traditional bleep

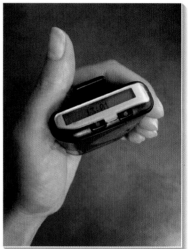

Source: *Courtesy of Camilla Thomas.*

**Figure 37.3** Prioritise jobs according to importance

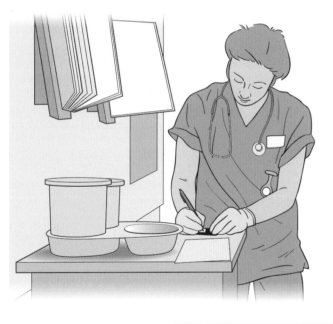

**Figure 37.4** Ensure that you eat, drink and take breaks

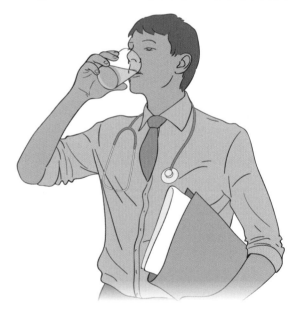

**Hints and Tips:**
- Ask for **help early**
- If in doubt, **ask!**
- Take regular breaks – eat, drink, rest
- Ask questions to the out-going juniors to facilitate a smooth transition and optimum care for the patients

There are now **compulsory shadowing periods** prior to the first 'real' day of being a doctor. Use this time to find out what will be expected of you, and how to meet those expectations. A new hospital, new people and new responsibilities can be both **exciting** and **daunting** – ensure that you focus on the actual **practicalities** of your work.

## Ward jobs

As a **junior doctor**, the responsibilities of preparing **patient ward lists** usually falls to you. Ward lists are surprisingly variable, with some Consultants preferring lists to be prepared in specific ways, while others are not so particular as long as you know where the patients are and what is going on with them. The ward lists are a **tool** for you to use, to ensure all patients are cared for properly (Figure 37.1). Find out how your new team do their ward lists, where these lists are saved on the computer directory and whether the team have any additional specifications that they like to have included. Along with the patient details, including ward name and bed number, the list usually includes admission date and reason, recent blood and other test results, and current management plans. Ensure that you know how to print this list, and ensure that you have enough copies ready for the upcoming ward rounds.

Use this patient ward list to note additional tests, results and management plan changes as they are mentioned **during** the **ward round**. Devise a system for marking on the list when actions have been started, completed or need to be 'chased'. Ensure that the actions are also recorded in the **patient's notes**. It can be useful for the junior doctors under the same Consultant to agree among themselves who will take on which role – who will write in the notes, who will read the observations, who will present the patient and who will record the additional tasks for the day on their ward list. Ensure that venous thromboembolism (VTE) assessments and prophylaxis are correctly documented and prescribed, respectively. Hospitals receive less funding if important aspects such as these are not documented adequately, even if the therapy has been delivered, so ensure that you know how and where to record this correctly.

This ward list will become your most prized possession. Fear will seep in at the thought of misplacing it, not only because of potential patient confidentiality breaches, but also for the indispensable information on current plans that it will contain. The ward list is like your **work plan** for the day.

Ensure that you become comfortable using **bleeps** at medical school (Figure 37.2). Each hospital will have a slightly different sequence of numbers and protocols. Find out your hospital's **important telephone numbers** and bleep numbers, how to **request investigations** – and where the food vending machines are! Keep your BNF and a clinical handbook handy at all times.

Familiarise yourself with **discharge planning** during your shadowing period. The main aim is for patients to be discharged home **swiftly** and **safely**. Ensure that you do not contribute to any delay in this process by understanding the timelines that are required by other members of the discharge team, such as Pharmacists. Remember that dosset boxes can take a few days to prepare, so organise these in advance. And remember that controlled drugs usually need to be prescribed differently from other medications (see Chapter 28).

## On-call jobs

Your first on-call will be an experience like no other – particularly your first night. You will be responsible for many **more patients**, with less support, than during your 'normal' ward job.

Ensure that you know how to contact your senior doctor, the **registrars** and the **on-call consultant**. Ensure you know how to request and access investigations. Ensure that you **answer bleeps promptly** – the one time that you do not, it will be a very sick patient.

On-calls can, at times, have a sense of 'fire-fighting' about them. Being **organised** and **prioritising appropriately** can help with this (Figure 37.3). **Write down all jobs** as they are given to you, with the time you received it, the extension number it was from, and devise a system for showing the actions you have taken. Ensure that this is clear, so that when you **hand over** at the end of your shift, you can easily identify which tasks still need doing or which results need checking. **Handover** is a key part of continuing patient care – ensure you know to which person you will handover, when and where to do this, and that you provide enough detail for each patient to be well cared for.

It can help to let the ward staff know in advance that you will come to their ward at a certain time, and asking them to prepare a list of **non-urgent requests** that you will see to at that time. This can mean fewer bleeps interrupting you while you perform other, more urgent jobs.

When bleeped about a **sick patient**, ensure that you remember to ask basic questions such as what the **observations** are – and do not forget the **patient's name** and **ward location**. In the initial rushes of adrenaline, these facts can be missed and only recalled after the call has ended! It can be helpful to ask for a repeat set of observations, an ECG and repeat bloods (if protocols permit) to be taken while you are on your way there, if this is clinically indicated. If the patient sounds very unwell, or there are several patients to see, ask for the nurse to bleep your senior or put out a crash call also.

## Breaks

When you feel as if there are too many things to do in too few hours, you may be tempted to put your own needs last. Food, drink and bathroom breaks vanish in the effort to save a few precious minutes. However, these economies are false, and you will be more **effective**, **efficient** and **competent** if you eat, drink and rest as needed. Take a break every 4 hours for 30 minutes (Figure 37.4).

## Asking for help

Remember that everyone had a first day. Do not feel ashamed to **ask for help**, particularly in the beginning. It is better to ask for help than to let a patient suffer.

Ensure that you have the **contact details** of key team members, including the **Medical Registrar**, at the start of any shift. When asking for help from them, ensure that you have key details, such as:

• Patient identification – name, date of birth, age, hospital number, ward, bed
• Current observations
• Patient history – admission details, treatment and investigations details, medications
• Current examination findings
• Current concerns.

Remember to keep **calm**, and **act professionally**, as you are a doctor now. Your diligence during medical school will have prepared you well.

**Good luck!**

# Further reading

Numerous resources were consulted during the preparation of this text. You will employ many more during your journey through medical school. Remember that resources that are recommended by your medical school have been recommended for a reason, such as for suitability in relation to depth and quality.

Reading widely facilitates your learning. You can broaden your perspectives on medical issues through reading books written by doctors, such as Atul Gawande and Ben Goldacre. Perusing primary literature will ensure that you keep aware of developments in current practice.

## General reading

Resources used in this book, or recommended generally, include:

British Medical Association: www.bma.org.uk [accessed on 8 August 2016].

General Medical Council: www.gmc-uk.org [accessed on 8 August 2016].

National Institute for Health and Care Excellence: www.nice.org.uk [accessed on 8 August 2016].

*At a Glance* series, Wiley-Blackwell, for example:

Blundell A., Harrison H. (2012) *OSCEs at a Glance*, 2nd edn. Wiley-Blackwell, Oxford.

Carney S., Gallen D. (2014) *The Foundation Programme at a Glance*. Wiley-Blackwell, Oxford.

Davey P. (2014) *Medicine at a Glance*, 4th edn. Wiley-Blackwell, Oxford.

Gleadle J. (2012) *History and Examination at a Glance*, 3rd edn. Wiley-Blackwell, Oxford.

Grace P.A., Borley N.R. (2013) *Surgery at a Glance*, 5th edn. Wiley-Blackwell, Oxford.

Thomas R.K. (2015) *Practical Medical Procedures at a Glance*. Wiley-Blackwell, Oxford.

Ward J.P., Linden R.W. (2013) *Physiology at a Glance*, 3rd edn. Wiley-Blackwell, Oxford.

*Oxford Handbook* series, Oxford University Press, for example:

Longmore M., Wilkinson I.B., Baldwin A., Wallin E. (2014) *Oxford Handbook of Clinical Medicine*, 9th edn. Oxford University Press, Oxford.

Raine T., McGinn K., Dawson J., et al. (2011) *Oxford Handbook for the Foundation Programme*, 3rd edn. Oxford University Press, Oxford.

Wilkins R., Cross S., Megson I., Meredith D. (2011) *Oxford Handbook of Medical Sciences*, 2nd edn. Oxford University Press, Oxford.

*Lecture Notes* series, Wiley-Blackwell, for example:

Ellis H., Calne R., Watson C. (2013) *Lecture Notes: General Surgery*, 12th edn. Wiley-Blackwell, Oxford.

*Essentials* series, Wiley-Blackwell, Oxford.

*Clinical Cases Uncovered* series, Wiley-Blackwell, Oxford.

*Kumar and Clark* series, Saunders, for example:

Ballinger A., Patchett S. (2008) *Kumar and Clark's Family Pocket Essentials of Clinical Medicine*, 4th edn. Saunders Elsevier, Edinburgh.

Franklin I., Dawson P.M. (2008) *Kumar and Clark's Family Pocket Essentials of Clinical Surgery*. Saunders Elsevier, Edinburgh.

Kumar P., Clark M.L. (2012) *Kumar and Clark's Clinical Medicine*, 8th edn. Saunders Elsevier, Edinburgh.

*Rapid* series, Wiley-Blackwell, for example:

Baker C.R., Reese G., Teo J.T. (2010) *Rapid Surgery*, 2nd edn. Wiley-Blackwell, Oxford.

Sam A.H., Teo J.T. (2010) *Rapid Medicine*, 2nd edn. Wiley Blackwell, Oxford.

Browse N., Black J., Burnand K., Thomas W. (2005) *Browse's Introduction to the Symptoms and Signs of Surgical Disease*, 4th edn. Hodder Arnold, London.

Dev H., Metcalfe D., Sanders S. (2014) *So You Want to Be a Doctor?* 2nd edn. Oxford University Press, Oxford.

Evans D., Brown J. (2009) *How to Succeed at Medical School*. Wiley-Blackwell, Oxford.

MacKinnon P., Morris M. (2005) *Oxford Textbook of Functional Anatomy*, vols 1, 2, 3. Oxford University Press, Oxford.

The following resources are particularly relevant in the individual chapters.

## Chapter 1 Starting medical school

Davey P. (2014) *Medicine at a Glance*, 4th edn. Wiley-Blackwell, Oxford.

Dev H., Metcalfe D., Sanders S. (2014) *So You Want to Be a Doctor?* 2nd edn. Oxford University Press, Oxford.

Faiz O., Moffat D. (2006) *Anatomy at a Glance*, 2nd edn. Wiley-Blackwell, Oxford.

General Medical Council: www.gmc-uk.org [accessed on 8 August 2016].

## Chapter 2 Medicine and surgery

Baker C.R, Reese G., Teo J.T. (2010) *Rapid Surgery*, 2nd edn. Wiley-Blackwell, Oxford.

Browse N., Black J., Burnand K., Thomas W. (2005) *Browse's Introduction to the Symptoms and Signs of Surgical Disease*, 4th edn. Hodder Arnold, London.

Carney S., Gallen D. (2014) *The Foundation Programme at a Glance*. Wiley-Blackwell, Oxford.

Collier J., Longmore M., Turmezei T., Mafi A. (2008) *Oxford Handbook of Clinical Specialities*, 8th edn. Oxford University Press, Oxford.

Dev H., Metcalfe D., Sanders S. (2014) *So You Want to Be a Doctor?* 2nd edn. Oxford University Press, Oxford.

Ellis H., Calne R., Watson C. (2011) *Lecture Notes: General Surgery*, 12th edn. Wiley Blackwell, Oxford.

Franklin I., Dawson P.M. (2008) *Kumar and Clark's Family Pocket Essentials of Clinical Surgery*. Saunders Elsevier, Edinburgh.

General Medical Council. Professionalism in action: http://www.gmc-uk.org/guidance/good_medical_practice/professionalism_in_action.asp [accessed on 8 August 2016].

NHS England. MTD delevopment: http://www.england.nhs.uk/wp-content/uploads/2015/01/mdt-dev-guid-flat-fin.pdf [accessed on 8 August 2016].

Sam A.H., Teo J.T. (2010) *Rapid Medicine*, 2nd edn. Wiley Blackwell, Oxford.

## Chapter 3 Understanding medical training

Admissions Testing Service. BioMedical Admissions Test (BMAT): http://www.admissionstestingservice.org/for-test-takers/bmat [accessed on 8 August 2016].

Carney S., Gallen D. (2014) *The Foundation Programme at a Glance*. Wiley-Blackwell, Oxford.

Collier J., Longmore M., Turmezei T., Mafi A. (2008) *Oxford Handbook of Clinical Specialities*, 8th edn. Oxford University Press, Oxford.

Dev H., Metcalfe D., Sanders S. (2014) *So You Want to Be a Doctor?* 2nd edn. Oxford University Press, Oxford.

Foundation Programme. About the programme: http://www.foundationprogramme.nhs.uk/pages/home/about-the-foundation-programme [accessed on 8 August 2016].

GAMSAT: www.gamsat.co.uk [accessed on 8 August 2016].

General Medical Council: www.gmc-uk.org [accessed on 8 August 2016].

Medical Schools Council. BMAT and UKCAT: http://www.medschools.ac.uk/Students/howtoapply/Pages/BMAT-and-UKCAT.aspx [accessed on 8 August 2016].

Medical Schools Council. UK Foundation Programme: http://www.medschools.ac.uk/Students/Pages/UK-Foundation-Programme.aspx [accessed on 8 August 2016].

NHS Health Careers. Medical specialty training: http://www.nhscareers.nhs.uk/explore-by-career/doctors/specialty-training/ [accessed on 8 August 2016].

NHS Health Education England. Health Education Thames Valley Recruitment 2016: FAQs: http://www.oxforddeanery.nhs.uk/recruitment__careers/hetv_recruitment_2014/recruitment_2014_faqs.aspx [accessed on 8 August 2016].

Raine T., McGinn K., Dawson J., et al. (2011) *Oxford Handbook for the Foundation Programme*, 3rd edn. Oxford University Press, Oxford.

UK Clinical Aptitude Test. Test format: http://www.ukcat.ac.uk/about-the-test/test-format/ [accessed on 8 August 2016].

## Chapter 4 Different learning mechanisms

British National Formulary: www.bnf.org [accessed on 8 August 2016].

Cochrane Collaboration: http://uk.cochrane.org [accessed on 8 August 2016].

Davey P. (2014) *Medicine at a Glance*, 4th edn. Wiley-Blackwell, Oxford.

Dev H., Metcalfe D., Sanders S. (2014) *So You Want to Be a Doctor?* 2nd edn. Oxford University Press, Oxford.

Evans D., Brown J. (2009) *How to Succeed at Medical School*. Wiley-Blackwell, Oxford.

National Institute for Health and Care Excellence: https://www.nice.org.uk/guidance [accessed on 8 August 2016].

PubMed: http://www.ncbi.nlm.nih.gov/pubmed [accessed on 8 August 2016].

## Chapter 5 Dealing with stress

British Medical Association: www.bma.org.uk [accessed on 8 August 2016].

Carney S., Gallen D. (2014) *The Foundation Programme at a Glance*. Wiley-Blackwell, Oxford.

General Medical Council: www.gmc-uk.org [accessed on 8 August 2016].

Raine T., McGinn K., Dawson J., et al. (2011) *Oxford Handbook for the Foundation Programme*, 3rd edn. Oxford University Press, Oxford.

World Health Organization. The ICD-10 Classification of Mental and Behavioural Disorders: http://www.who.int/classifications/icd/en/bluebook.pdf [accessed on 8 August 2016].

## Chapter 6 Solving issues

British Medical Association: www.bma.org.uk [accessed on 8 August 2016].

General Medical Council: www.gmc-uk.org [accessed on 8 August 2016].

Medical Defence Union: www.themdu.com [accessed on 8 August 2016].

Medical Protection Society: www.medicalprotection.org.uk [accessed on 8 August 2016].

Tasker F. How to lead a quality improvement project: http://careers.bmj.com/careers/advice/view-article.html?id=20010482 [accessed on 8 August 2016].

## Chapter 7 Important common principles

Ballinger A., Patchett S. (2008) *Kumar and Clark's Family Pocket Essentials of Clinical Medicine*, 4th edn. Saunders Elsevier, Edinburgh.

Davey P. (2014) *Medicine at a Glance*, 4th edn. Wiley-Blackwell, Oxford.

Department of Health: https://www.gov.uk/government/organisations/department-of-health [accessed on 8 August 2016].

Franklin I., Dawson P.M. (2008) *Kumar and Clark's Family Pocket Essentials of Clinical Surgery*. Saunders Elsevier, Edinburgh.

General Medical Council: www.gmc-uk.org [accessed on 8 August 2016].

Gleadle J. (2012) *History and Examination at a Glance*, 3rd edn. Wiley-Blackwell, Oxford.

Health and Safety Executive. Control of Substances Hazardous to Health (COSHH): www.hse.gov.uk/coshh/ [accessed on 8 August 2016].

Hope T., Savulescu J., Hendrick J. (2003) *Medical Ethics and the Law: The Core Curriculum*. Churchill Livingstone, Elsevier.

NHS England. Never Events List 2015/16: https://www.england.nhs.uk/wp-content/uploads/2015/03/never-evnts-list-15-16.pdf [accessed on 8 August 2016].

Thomas R.K. (2015) *Practical Medical Procedures at a Glance*. Wiley-Blackwell, Oxford.

World Health Organization: www.who.int [accessed on 8 August 2016].

## Chapter 8 Ethics

Ballinger A., Patchett S. (2008) *Kumar and Clark's Family Pocket Essentials of Clinical Medicine*, 4th edn. Saunders Elsevier, Edinburgh.

Beauchamp T., Childress J. (2001) *Principles Biomedical Ethics*, 5th edn. Oxford University Press, Oxford.

British Medical Association. Ethics: bma.org.uk/ethics [accessed on 8 August 2016].

Clinical Ethics Network: http://www.ukcen.net/index.php/ ethical_issues/ethical_frameworks/the_four_principles_of_ biomedical_ethics [accessed on 8 August 2016].

Davey P. (2014) *Medicine at a Glance*, 4th edn. Wiley-Blackwell, Oxford.

General Medical Council: www.gmc-uk.org [accessed on 8 August 2016].

Hope T., Savulescu J., Hendrick J. (2003) *Medical Ethics and the Law: The Core Curriculum*. Churchill Livingstone, Elsevier.

*Journal of Medical Ethics*: http://jme.bmj.com [accessed on 8 August 2016].

Longmore M., Wilkinson I.B., Baldwin A., Wallin E. (2014) *Oxford Handbook of Clinical Medicine*, 9th edn. Oxford University Press, Oxford.

Raine T., McGinn K., Dawson J., et al. (2011) *Oxford Handbook for the Foundation Programme*, 3rd edn. Oxford University Press, Oxford.

Royal College of Nursing. Dignity: https://www.rcn.org.uk/__data/ assets/pdf_file/0003/191730/003298.pdf [accessed on 8 August 2016].

Sokol DK. 'First do no harm' revisited. *BMJ* 2013;347:f6426: http:// www.bmj.com/content/347/bmj.f6426 [accessed on 8 August 2016].

## Chapter 9 Communication skills and teamwork

Blundell A., Harrison H. (2012) *OSCEs at a Glance*, 2nd edn. Wiley-Blackwell, Oxford.

Carney S., Gallen D. (2014) *The Foundation Programme at a Glance*. Wiley-Blackwell, Oxford.

Donald A., Stein M., Scott Hill C. (2011) *The Hands-on Guide for Junior Doctors*, 4th edn. Wiley-Blackwell, Oxford.

Evans D., Brown J. (2009) *How to Succeed at Medical School*. Wiley-Blackwell, Oxford.

General Medical Council: www.gmc-uk.org [accessed on 8 August 2016].

Gleadle J. (2012) *History and Examination at a Glance*, 3rd edn. Wiley-Blackwell, Oxford.

Longmore M., Wilkinson I.B., Baldwin A., Wallin E. (2014) *Oxford Handbook of Clinical Medicine*, 9th edn. Oxford University Press, Oxford.

Patient: www.patient.co.uk [accessed on 8 August 2016].

Raine T., McGinn K., Dawson J., et al. (2011) *Oxford Handbook for the Foundation Programme*, 3rd edn. Oxford University Press, Oxford.

Thomas J., Monaghan T. (2010) *Oxford Handbook of Clinical Examination and Practical Skills*. Oxford University Press, Oxford.

Thomas R.K. (2015) *Practical Medical Procedures at a Glance*. Wiley-Blackwell, Oxford.

## Chapter 10 Balance

Carney S., Gallen D. (2014) *The Foundation Programme at a Glance*. Wiley-Blackwell, Oxford.

Evans D., Brown J. (2009) *How to Succeed at Medical School*. Wiley-Blackwell, Oxford.

## Chapter 11 Evidence-based medicine

Belsey J., Snell T. (2009) What is evidence-based medicine? http:// www.medicine.ox.ac.uk/bandolier/painres/download/whatis/ ebm.pdf [accessed on 8 August 2016].

Benjamin A. (2008) Audit: how to do it in practice. *BMJ* 336:1241– 1245.

BMJ. Statistics at Square One: http://www.bmj.com/about-bmj/ resources-readers/publications/statistics-square-one [accessed on 8 August 2016]

Carney S., Gallen D. (2014) *The Foundation Programme at a Glance*. Wiley-Blackwell, Oxford.

Centre for Evidence-Based Medicine: http://www.cebm.net/ oxford-centre-evidence-based-medicine-levels-evidence-march-2009/ [accessed on 8 August 2016].

Cochrane Collaboration: http://uk.cochrane.org [accessed on 8 August 2016].

Cochrane Library Tutorial. Medical literature searching skills: http://learntech.physiol.ox.ac.uk/cochrane_tutorial/ cochlibd0e84.php [accessed on 8 August 2016].

Donald A., Stein M., Scott Hill C. (2011) *The Hands-on Guide for Junior Doctors*, 4th edn. Wiley-Blackwell, Oxford.

E Medicine: www.emedicine.com [accessed on 8 August 2016].

EBM Pyramid, Produced by Jan Glover, David Izzo, Karen Odato and Lei Wang copyright 2006 Trustees of Dartmouth College and Yale University. http://guides.nnlm.gov/content. php?pid=366644&sid=3399389 [accessed on 8 August 2016].

Greenhalgh T. (2010) *How to Read a Paper: The Basics of Evidence-based Medicine*, 4th edn. Wiley-Blackwell, Oxford.

Greenhalgh T., Howick J., Maskrey N. (2014) Evidence Based Medicine Renaissance Group. Evidence based medicine: a movement in crisis? *BMJ* 348:g3725.

Longmore M., Wilkinson I.B., Baldwin A., Wallin E. (2014) *Oxford Handbook of Clinical Medicine*, 9th edn. Oxford University Press, Oxford.

NHS evidence: www.evidence.nhs.uk [accessed on 8 August 2016].

Oxford Centre for Evidence-based Medicine: http://www.cebm. net/oxford-centre-evidence-based-medicine-levels-evidence-march-2009/ [accessed on 8 August 2016].

Patient info: http://patient.info/doctor/Audit-and-Audit-Cycle#ref-1. [accessed on 8 August 2016].

Patient info: http://patient.info/doctor/different-levels-of-evidence. [accessed on 8 August 2016].

Petrie A., Sabin C. (2009) *Medical Statistics at a Glance*. Wiley-Blackwell, Oxford.

Raine T., McGinn K., Dawson J., et al. (2011) *Oxford Handbook for the Foundation Programme*, 3rd edn. Oxford University Press, Oxford.

Rosenberg W., Donald A. (1995) Evidence based medicine: an approach to clinical problem solving. *BMJ* 310:1122–1126.

Sackett D.L., Rosenberg W.M., Gray J.A., et al. (1996) Evidence based medicine: what it is and what it isn't. *BMJ* 312:71–72.

University of Manchester. PEPS: Clinical Quality and Evidence: https://online.manchester.ac.uk/bbcswebdav/orgs/I3075-COMMUNITY-MEDN-1/DO%20NOT%20DELETE%20 -%20PEP%20Quality%20and%20Evidence/QE-PEP-HTML5/ AN-232E8560-4F14-1254-C272-DE02E63DB32D.html [accessed on 8 August 2016].

## Chapter 12 Understanding guidelines

Carney S., Gallen D. (2014) *The Foundation Programme at a Glance*. Wiley-Blackwell, 2014.

Cochrane Collaboration: http://uk.cochrane.org [accessed on 8 August 2016].

eMedicine: www.emedicine.com [accessed on 8 August 2016].

General Medical Council: www.gmc-uk.org [accessed on 8 August 2016].

Guidance from NICE: https://www.nice.org.uk/guidance [accessed on 8 August 2016].

Guidelines: www.guidelines.co.uk/ [accessed on 8 August 2016].

Resuscitation Council (UK): www.resus.org.uk/ [accessed on 8 August 2016].

## Chapter 13 Behaving on the ward

Carney S., Gallen D. (2014) *The Foundation Programme at a Glance.* Wiley-Blackwell, Oxford.

Davey P. (2014) *Medicine at a Glance*, 4th edn. Wiley-Blackwell, Oxford.

General Medical Council: www.gmc-uk.org [accessed on 8 August 2016].

Gleadle J. (2012) *History and Examination at a Glance*, 3rd edn. Wiley-Blackwell, Oxford.

Longmore M., Wilkinson I.B., Baldwin A., Wallin E. (2014) *Oxford Handbook of Clinical Medicine*, 9th edn. Oxford University Press, Oxford.

Raine T., McGinn K., Dawson J., et al. (2011) *Oxford Handbook for the Foundation Programme*, 3rd edn. Oxford University Press, Oxford.

## Chapter 14 Behaving in theatre

General Medical Council: www.gmc-uk.org [accessed on 8 August 2016].

NHS. How to guide to the five steps to safer surgery NHS Direct, 2010: http://www.nrls.npsa.nhs.uk/resources/?EntryId45=92901 [accessed on 8 August 2016].

NHS. Patient Safety Alert – WHO Surgical Safety Checklist, 2009: http://www.nrls.npsa.nhs.uk/resources/clinical-specialty/surgery/ [accessed on 8 August 2016].

NHS. Safer Practice Notice – Standardising wristbands improves patient safety, 2007: http://www.nrls.npsa.nhs.uk/resources/?entryid45=59824 [accessed on 8 August 2016].

Raine T., McGinn K., Dawson J., et al. (2011) *Oxford Handbook for the Foundation Programme*, 3rd edn. Oxford University Press, Oxford.

Royal College of Anaesthetics. Guide for Novice Trainees: http://www.e-lfh.org.uk/e-learning-sessions/rcoa-novice/content/home/tips.html [accessed on 8 August 2016].

Royal College of Ophthalmologists. Safer Surgery Checklist for Cataract Surgery, 2010: https://www.rcophth.ac.uk/wp-content/uploads/2014/12/2010-SCI-069-Cataract-Surgery-Guidelines-2010-SEPTEMBER-2010.pdf [accessed on 8 August 2016].

Uckay I., Harbarth S., Peter R., et al. (2010) Preventing surgical site infections. *Expert Rev Anti Infect Ther* 8(6):657–670. www.medscape.com/viewarticle/723601_4 [accessed on 8 August 2016].

World Health Organization. Surgical Safety Checklist: https://atpbio.files.wordpress.com/2013/04/surgical-safety-checklist-who.jpg [accessed on 8 August 2016].

## Chapter 15 Behaving in clinic

Evans D., Brown J. (2009) *How to Succeed at Medical School: An Essential Guide to Learning.* Wiley-Blackwell, Oxford.

General Medical Council. Intimate examinations and chaperones (2013): http://www.gmc-uk.org/guidance/ethical_guidance/21168.asp [accessed on 8 August 2016].

Gleadle J. (2012) *History and Examination at a Glance*, 3rd edn. Wiley-Blackwell, Oxford.

## Chapter 16 Learning practical procedures

Al-Elq A.H. (2010) Simulation-based medical teaching and learning. *J Family Community Med* 17(1):35–40. doi: 10.4103/1319-1683.68787 [accessed on 8 August 2016].

Blundell A., Harrison H. (2012) *OSCEs at a Glance*, 2nd edn. Wiley-Blackwell, Oxford.

Carney S., Gallen D. (2014) *The Foundation Programme at a Glance.* Wiley-Blackwell, Oxford.

Department of Health. The never events policy framework: https://www.gov.uk/government/uploads/system/uploads/attachment_data/file/213046/never-events-policy-framework-update-to-policy.pdf [accessed on 8 August 2016].

Donald A., Stein M., Scott Hill C. (2011) *The Hands-on Guide for Junior Doctors*, 4th edn. Wiley-Blackwell, Oxford.

Franklin I., Dawson P.M. (2008) *Kumar and Clark's Family Pocket Essentials of Clinical Surgery.* Saunders Elsevier, Edinburgh.

General Medical Council: www.gmc-uk.org [accessed on 8 August 2016].

Health and Safety Executive. Control of Substances Hazardous to Health: www.hse.gov.uk/coshh/ [accessed on 8 August 2016].

Jabbar Ul., Leischner J., Kasper D., et al. (2010) Effectiveness of alcohol-based hand rubs for removal of *Clostridium difficile* spores from hands. *Infect Control Hosp Epidemiol* 31(6):565–570. doi: 10.1086/652772 [accessed on 8 August 2016].

Longmore M., Wilkinson I.B., Baldwin A., Wallin E. (2014) *Oxford Handbook of Clinical Medicine*, 9th edn. Oxford University Press, Oxford.

National Patient Safety Association. Core list of Never Events: http://www.nrls.npsa.nhs.uk/resources/collections/never-events/core-list/ [accessed on 8 August 2016].

NHS England. Never Events List 2015/16. http://www.england.nhs.uk/wp-content/uploads/2015/03/never-evnts-list-15-16.pdf [accessed on 8 August 2016].

Raine T., McGinn K., Dawson J., et al. (2011) *Oxford Handbook for the Foundation Programme*, 3rd edn. Oxford University Press, Oxford.

Stephenson M., Shur J., Black J. (2013) *How to Perform Clinical Procedures.* Wiley-Blackwell, Oxford.

Thomas J., Monaghan T. (2010) *Oxford Handbook of Clinical Examination and Practical Skills.* Oxford University Press, Oxford.

Thomas R.K. (2015) *Practical Medical Procedures at a Glance.* Wiley-Blackwell, Oxford.

## Chapter 17 Approaching a patient

Blundell A., Harrison, H. (2012) *OSCEs at a Glance*, 2nd edn. Wiley-Blackwell, Oxford.

Davey P. (2014) *Medicine at a Glance*, 4th edn. Wiley-Blackwell, Oxford.

General Medical Council: www.gmc-uk.org [accessed on 8 August 2016].

Gleadle J. (2012) *History and Examination at a Glance*, 3rd edn. Wiley-Blackwell, Oxford.

Raine T., McGinn K., Dawson J., et al. (2011) *Oxford Handbook for the Foundation Programme*, 3rd edn. Oxford University Press, Oxford.

Thomas R.K. (2015) *Practical Medical Procedures at a Glance.* Wiley-Blackwell, Oxford.

## Chapter 18 Approaching an unwell patient

Blundell A., Harrison H. (2012) *OSCEs at a Glance*, 2nd edn. Wiley-Blackwell, Oxford.

Carney S., Gallen D. (2014) *The Foundation Programme at a Glance*. Wiley-Blackwell, Oxford.

Davey P. (2014) *Medicine at a Glance*, 4th edn. Wiley-Blackwell, Oxford.

Franklin I., Dawson P.M. (2008) *Kumar and Clark's Family Pocket Essentials of Clinical Surgery*. Saunders Elsevier, Edinburgh.

Leach R.M. (2014) *Critical Care Medicine at a Glance*, 3rd edn. Wiley-Blackwell, Oxford.

Longmore M., Wilkinson I.B., Baldwin A., Wallin E. (2014) *Oxford Handbook of Clinical Medicine*, 9th edn. Oxford University Press, Oxford.

Raine T., McGinn K., Dawson J., et al. (2014) *Oxford Handbook for the Foundation Programme*, 3rd edn. Oxford University Press, Oxford.

Smith G. (2003) *ALERT Course Manual*. University of Portsmouth, UK.

Wyatt J., Illingworth R., Graham C., Hogg K. (2012) *Oxford Handbook of Emergency Medicine*, 4th edn. Oxford University Press, Oxford.

## Chapter 19 Taking a history

Blundell A., Harrison H. (2012) *OSCEs at a Glance*, 2nd edn. Wiley-Blackwell, 2012

Browse N., Black J., Burnand K., Thomas W. (2005) *Browse's Introduction to the Symptoms and Signs of Surgical Disease*, 4th edn. Hodder Arnold, London.

Chow J., Yvon C., Stanger T. (2014) How complete are our clerkings? A project aimed at improving the quality of medical records by using a standardised proforma. *BMJ Qual Improv Rep* 2:pii: http://qir.bmj.com/content/2/2/u203012.w1388.full.pdf [accessed on 8 August 2016].

Davey P. (2014) *Medicine at a Glance*, 4th edn. Wiley-Blackwell, Oxford.

Donald A., Stein M., Scott Hill C. (2011) *The Hands-on Guide for Junior Doctors*, 4th edn. Wiley-Blackwell, Oxford.

Drinkaware. Unit and calorie calculator: https://www.drinkaware.co.uk/understand-your-drinking/unit-calculator [accessed on 8 August 2016].

Gleadle J. (2012) *History and Examination at a Glance*, 3rd edn. Wiley-Blackwell, Oxford.

OSCE Skills. History taking: http://www.osceskills.com/e-learning/subjects/patient-history-taking/ [accessed on 8 August 2016].

Patient. History taking: http://patient.info/doctor/history-taking [accessed on 8 August 2016].

Raine T., McGinn K., Dawson J., et al. (2011) *Oxford Handbook for the Foundation Programme*, 3rd edn. Oxford University Press, Oxford.

Thomas J., Monaghan T. (2010) *Oxford Handbook of Clinical Examination and Practical Skills*. Oxford University Press, Oxford.

## Chapter 20 Examining a patient

Blundell A., Harrison H. (2012) *OSCEs at a Glance*, 2nd edn. Wiley-Blackwell, Oxford.

Browse N., Black J., Burnand K., Thomas W. (2005) *Browse's Introduction to the Symptoms and Signs of Surgical Disease*, 4th edn. Hodder Arnold, London.

Davey P. (2014) *Medicine at a Glance*, 4th edn. Wiley-Blackwell, Oxford.

General Medical Council: www.gmc-uk.org [accessed on 8 August 2016].

Gleadle J. (2012) *History and Examination at a Glance*, 3rd edn. Wiley-Blackwell, Oxford.

Raine T., McGinn K., Dawson J., et al. (2011) *Oxford Handbook for the Foundation Programme*, 3rd edn. Oxford University Press, Oxford.

Thomas J., Monaghan T. (2010) *Oxford Handbook of Clinical Examination and Practical Skills*. Oxford University Press, Oxford.

## Chapter 21 Assessing a patient's hydration

Ballinger A., Patchett S. (2008) *Kumar and Clark's Family Pocket Essentials of Clinical Medicine*, 4th edn. Saunders Elsevier, Edinburgh.

Carney S., Gallen D. (2014) *The Foundation Programme at a Glance*. Wiley-Blackwell, Oxford.

Davey P. (2014) *Medicine at a Glance*, 4th edn. Wiley-Blackwell, Oxford.

Gleadle J. (2012) *History and Examination at a Glance*, 3rd edn. Wiley-Blackwell, Oxford.

Raine T., McGinn K., Dawson J., et al. (2011) *Oxford Handbook for the Foundation Programme*, 3rd edn. Oxford University Press, Oxford.

## Chapter 22 Assessing a patient's nutrition

Carney S., Gallen D. (2014) *The Foundation Programme at a Glance*. Wiley-Blackwell, Oxford.

Davey P. (2014) *Medicine at a Glance*, 4th edn. Wiley-Blackwell, Oxford.

Gleadle J. (2012) *History and Examination at a Glance*, 3rd edn. Wiley-Blackwell, Oxford.

Mehanna H.M., Moledina J., Travis J. (2008) Refeeding syndrome: what it is, and how to prevent and treat it. *BMJ* 336:1495–1498: http://www.ncbi.nlm.nih.gov/pmc/articles/PMC2440847 [accessed on 8 August 2016]

Raine T., McGinn K., Dawson J., et al. (2011) *Oxford Handbook for the Foundation Programme*, 3rd edn. Oxford University Press, Oxford.

Royal College of Physicians. Nutrition – top ten tips: https://www.rcplondon.ac.uk/projects/outputs/nutrition-top-ten-tips [accessed on 8 August 2016].

## Chapter 23 Investigations

Blundell A., Harrison H. (2012) *OSCEs at a Glance*, 2nd edn. Wiley-Blackwell, Oxford.

General Medical Council: www.gmc-uk.org [accessed on 8 August 2016].

Raine T., McGinn K., Dawson J., et al. (2011) *Oxford Handbook for the Foundation Programme*, 3rd edn. Oxford University Press, Oxford.

Weir J., Abrahams P.H., Belli A., et al. (2003) *Imaging Atlas of Human Anatomy*, 3rd edn. Mosby, Elsevier.

## Chapter 24 Considering diagnoses

American Medical Association: www.ama-assn.org [accessed on 8 August 2016].

Barondess J.A., Carpenter C.C.J. (eds). (1994) *Differential Diagnosis*. Lea & Febiger, Philadelphia.

Davey P. (2014) *Medicine at a Glance*, 4th edn. Wiley-Blackwell, Oxford.

Gleadle J. (2012) *History and Examination at a Glance*, 3rd edn. Wiley-Blackwell, Oxford.

Johns Hopkins Arthritis Center. ACR Diagnostic Guidelines: http://www.hopkinsarthritis.org/physician-corner/education/

arthritis-education-diagnostic-guidelines/ [accessed on 8 August 2016].

Raftery A.T., Lim E. (2008) *Churchill's Pocketbooks Differential Diagnosis.* Elsevier Churchill Livingstone, Elsevier.

Ramrakha P.S., Moore K.P., Sam A. (2010) *Oxford Handbook of Acute Medicine*, 3rd edn. Oxford University Press, Oxford.

Richardson W.S., Wilson M., Guyatt G. (2002) The process of diagnosis. *The American Medical Association.* http://medicine. ucsf.edu/education/resed/articles/jama6_the_process.pdf [accessed on 8 August 2016].

Turmezei T. (2009) The surgical sieve. *BMJ* 339:b5384: http://www. bmj.com/content/339/bmj.b5384 [accessed on 8 August 2016].

UpToDate. Differential diagnosis of chect pain in adults: http://www.uptodate.com/contents/differential-diagnosis-of-chest-pain-in-adults [accessed on 8 August 2016].

## Chapter 25 Presenting a patient

Blundell A., Harrison H. (2012) *OSCEs at a Glance*, 2nd edn. Wiley-Blackwell, Oxford.

Davey P. (2014) *Medicine at a Glance*, 4th edn. Wiley-Blackwell, Oxford.

Gleadle J. (2012) *History and Examination at a Glance*, 3rd edn. Wiley-Blackwell, Oxford.

Longmore M., Wilkinson I.B., Baldwin A., Wallin E. (2014) *Oxford Handbook of Clinical Medicine*, 9th edn. Oxford University Press, Oxford.

Olaitan O., Lkunade O., Corne J. How to present clinical cases. *Student BMJ:* http://student.bmj.com/student/view-article. html?id=id:5136 [accessed on 8 August 2016].

## Chapter 26 Consent and capacity

Blundell A., Harrison H. (2012) *OSCEs at a Glance*, 2nd edn. Wiley-Blackwell, Oxford.

Carney S., Gallen D. (2014) *The Foundation Programme at a Glance.* Wiley-Blackwell, Oxford.

Davey P. (2014) *Medicine at a Glance*, 4th edn. Wiley-Blackwell, Oxford.

Donald A., Stein M., Scott Hill C. (2011) *The Hands-on Guide for Junior Doctors*, 4th edn. Wiley-Blackwell, Oxford.

General Medical Council. Consent: patients and doctors making decisions together: http://www.gmc-uk.org/guidance/ethical_ guidance/consent_guidance_index.asp [accessed on 8 August 2016].

General Medical Council. Consent guidance: Legal Annex – Common Law: www.gponline.com/medico-legal-gillick-competence/article/1057179 [accessed on 8 August 2016].

Gleadle J. (2012) *History and Examination at a Glance*, 3rd edn. Wiley-Blackwell, Oxford.

Katona C., Cooper C., Robertson M. (2015) *Psychiatry at a Glance*, 5th edn. Wiley-Blackwell, Oxford.

Mental Capacity Act 2005: http://www.legislation.gov.uk/ ukpga/2005/9/contents [accessed on 8 August 2016].

NHS. *What is the Mental Capacity Act?* http://www.nhs.uk/ conditions/social-care-and-support-guide/pages/mental-capacity.aspx [accessed on 8 August 2016].

NSPCC. Gillick competency and Fraser guidelines: www.nspcc. org.uk [accessed on 8 August 2016].

Raine T., McGinn K., Dawson J., et al. (2011) *Oxford Handbook for the Foundation Programme*, 3rd edn. Oxford University Press, Oxford.

Semple D., Smyth R. (2010) *Oxford Handbook of Psychiatry*, 2nd edn. Oxford University Press, Oxford.

## Chapter 27 Breaking bad news

Adler D.D., Riba M.B., Eggly S. (2009) Breaking bad news in the breast imaging setting. *Acad Radiol* 16(2):130–135

Baile W.F., Buckman R., Lenzi R., et al. (2000) SPIKES: A six-step protocol for delivering bad news: application to the patient with cancer. *Oncologist* 5(4):302–311.

Blundell A., Harrison H. (2012) *OSCEs at a Glance*, 2nd edn. Wiley-Blackwell, Oxford.

BMA: www.bma.org.uk [accessed on 8 August 2016].

Carney S., Gallen D. (2014) *The Foundation Programme at a Glance.* Wiley-Blackwell, Oxford.

Department of Health, Social Services and Public Safety: www. Dhsspsni.gov.uk [accessed on 8 August 2016].

Donald A., Stein M., Scott Hill C. (2011) *The Hands-on Guide for Junior Doctors*, 4th edn. Wiley-Blackwell, Oxford.

General Medical Council: www.gmc-uk.org [accessed on 8 August 2016].

Longmore M., Wilkinson I.B., Baldwin A., Wallin E. (2014) *Oxford Handbook of Clinical Medicine*, 9th edn. Oxford University Press, Oxford.

Narayanan V., Bista B., Koshy C. (2010) 'BREAKS' protocol for breaking bad news. *Indian J Palliat Care* 16(2):61–65. doi: 10.4103/0973-1075.68401 [accessed on 8 August 2016].

Raine T., McGinn K., Dawson J., et al. (2011) *Oxford Handbook for the Foundation Programme*, 3rd edn. Oxford University Press, Oxford.

Skill cascade: www.Skillscascade.com [accessed on 8 August 2016].

## Chapter 28 Prescribing

Blundell A., Harrison H. (2012) *OSCEs at a Glance*, 2nd edn. Wiley-Blackwell, Oxford.

British Medical Association and the Royal Pharmaceutical Society (2013) published jointly by BMJ group and Pharmaceutical Press. *British National Formulary* 2013: www.bnf.org [accessed on 8 August 2016].

Carney S., Gallen D. (2014) *The Foundation Programme at a Glance.* Wiley-Blackwell, Oxford.

Donald A., Stein M., Scott Hill C. (2011) *The Hands-on Guide for Junior Doctors*, 4th edn. Wiley-Blackwell, Oxford.

General Medical Council: www.gmc-uk.org [accessed on 8 August 2016].

Neal M.J. (2009) *Medical Pharmacology at a Glance*, 7th edn. Wiley-Blackwell, Oxford.

Nicholson T.R., Singer D.R. (2016) *Pocket Prescriber 2015.* CRC Press, Florida.

Raine T., McGinn K., Dawson J., et al. (2011) *Oxford Handbook for the Foundation Programme*, 3rd edn. Oxford University Press, Oxford.

Richards D., Aronson J. (2011) *Oxford Handbook of Practical Drug Therapy.* Oxford University Press, Oxford.

## Chapter 29 Documentation

Carney S., Gallen D. (2014) *The Foundation Programme at a Glance.* Wiley-Blackwell, Oxford.

General Medical Council: www.gmc-uk.org [accessed on 8 August 2016].

Matin R.N.H. (2006) Writing clinical records ona consultant ward round. *BMA Careers,* http://careers.bmj.com/careers/advice/ view-article.html?id=1811 [accessed on 8 August 2016].

Raine T., McGinn K., Dawson J., et al. (2011) *Oxford Handbook for the Foundation Programme*, 3rd edn. Oxford University Press, Oxford.

## Chapter 30 Discharge planning

Carney S., Gallen D. (2014) *The Foundation Programme at a Glance*. Wiley-Blackwell, Oxford.

## Chapter 31 Managing the acutely unwell patient

Blundell A., Harrison H. (2012) *OSCEs at a Glance*, 2nd edn. Wiley-Blackwell, Oxford.

Browse N., Black J., Burnand K., Thomas W. (2005) *Browse's Introduction to the Symptoms and Signs of Surgical Disease*, 4th edn. Hodder Arnold, London.

Carney S., Gallen D. (2014) *The Foundation Programme at a Glance*. Wiley-Blackwell, Oxford.

Davey P. (2014) *Medicine at a Glance*, 4th edn. Wiley-Blackwell, Oxford.

Frost P.J. (2012) Early management of acutely ill ward patients. *BMJ* 345:e5677: http://www.bmj.com/content/345/bmj.e5677 [accessed on 8 August 2016]

Ramrakha P.S., Moore K.P., Sam A. (2010) *Oxford Handbook of Acute Medicine*, 3rd edn. Oxford University Press, Oxford.

Resuscitation Council UK. A systematic approach to the acutely ill patient (ABCDE approach): https://www.resus.org.uk/archive/guidelines-2010/a-systematic-approach-to-the-acutely-ill-patient-abcde/ [accessed on 8 August 2016]

Smith G. (2003) *ALERT Course Manual*. University of Portsmouth, UK.

Wyatt J., Illingworth R., Graham C., Hogg K. (2012) *Oxford Handbook of Emergency Medicine*, 4th edn. Oxford University Press, Oxford.

## Chapter 32 Examinations

Blundell A., Harrison H. (2012) *OSCEs at a Glance*, 2nd edn. Wiley-Blackwell, Oxford.

Browse N., Black J., Burnand K., Thomas W. (2005) *Browse's Introduction to the Symptoms and Signs of Surgical Disease*, 4th ed., Hodder Arnold, London.

Davey P. (2014) *Medicine at a Glance*, 4th edn. Wiley-Blackwell, Oxford.

Gleadle J. (2012) *History and Examination at a Glance*, 3rd edn. Wiley-Blackwell, Oxford.

## Chapter 33 Electives and special study modules

Evans D., Brown J. (2009) *How to Succeed at Medical School: An Essential Guide to Learning*. Wiley-Blackwell, Oxford.

Gleadle J. (2012) *History and Examination at a Glance*, 3rd edn. Wiley-Blackwell, Oxford.

Medical Schools Council. Electives: http://www.medschools.ac.uk/Students/electives/Pages/default.aspx [accessed on 8 August 2016].

## Chapter 34 Understanding foundation school

Academy of Medical Royal Colleges: www.aomrc.org.uk [accessed on 8 August 2016].

Carney S., Gallen D. (2014) *The Foundation Programme at a Glance*. Wiley-Blackwell, Oxford.

Evans D., Brown J. (2009) *How to Succeed at Medical School: An Essential Guide to Learning*. Wiley-Blackwell, Oxford.

Foundation Programme. FAQs: http://www.foundationprogramme.nhs.uk/pages/medical-students/faqs [accessed on 8 August 2016].

Longmore M., Wilkinson I.B., Baldwin A., Wallin E. (2014) *Oxford Handbook of Clinical Medicine*, 9th edn. Oxford University Press, Oxford.

Medical careers: www.medicalcareers.nhs.uk [accessed on 8 August 2016].

Raine T., McGinn K., Dawson J., et al. (2011) *Oxford Handbook for the Foundation Programme*, 3rd edn. Oxford University Press, Oxford.

Skills for health: www.skillsforhealth.org.uk [accessed on 8 August 2016].

## Chapter 35 Understanding later training

Carney S., Gallen D. (2014) *The Foundation Programme at a Glance*. Wiley-Blackwell, Oxford.

Collier J., Longmore M., Turmezei T., Mafi A. (2008) *Oxford Handbook of Clinical Specialities*, 8th edn. Oxford University Press, Oxford.

General Medical Council: www.gmc-uk.org [accessed on 8 August 2016].

Gold Guide. A reference guide for postgraduate specialty training in the UK: http://specialtytraining.hee.nhs.uk/files/2013/10/Gold-Guide-6th-Edition-February-2016.pdf [accessed on 8 August 2016].

NHS Health Education England. Specialty training programme information: https://www.eastmidlandsdeanery.nhs.uk/page.php?id=1527 [accessed on 8 August 2016].

Raine T., McGinn K., Dawson J., et al. (2011) *Oxford Handbook for the Foundation Programme*, 3rd edn. Oxford University Press, Oxford.

Simon C., Everitt H., Kendrick T. (2008) *Oxford Handbook of General Practice*, 2nd edn. Oxford University Press, Oxford.

## Chapter 36 Other uses for medical degrees

BMJ careers: http://careers.bmj.com [accessed on 8 August 2016].

NHS careers: https://www.healthcareers.nhs.uk/ [accessed on 8 August 2016].

## Chapter 37 First day as a doctor

British Medical Association. (2012) *BMA Junior Doctors' Handbook*. BMA, London.

Carney S., Gallen D. (2014) *The Foundation Programme at a Glance*. Wiley-Blackwell, Oxford.

Davey P. (2014) *Medicine at a Glance*, 4th edn. Wiley-Blackwell, Oxford.

Donald A., Stein M., Scott Hill C. (2011) *The Hands-on Guide for Junior Doctors*, 4th edn. Wiley-Blackwell, Oxford.

Gallen D., Buckle G. (1997) *Top Tips in Primary Care Management*. Blackwell Science, Oxford.

General Medical Council. Important information about provisional registration: http://www.gmc-uk.org/doctors/registration_applications/11720.asp [accessed on 8 August 2016].

Raine T., McGinn K., Dawson J., et al. (2011) *Oxford Handbook for the Foundation Programme*, 3rd edn. Oxford University Press, Oxford.

# Index